Obstetrics and Gynaecology

CLINICAL CASES UNCOVERED

Maggie Cruickshank
MBChB, MD, FRCOG
Senior Lecturer in Gynaecology
Aberdeen Maternity Hospital,
Foresterhill,
Aberdeen, UK

Ashalatha Shetty
MD, MRCOG, MRCP(I), DGO
Consultant in Obstetrics and Fetal–Maternal Medicine
Aberdeen Maternity Hospital,
Foresterhill,
Aberdeen, UK

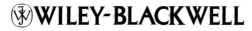
WILEY-BLACKWELL

A John Wiley & Sons. Ltd.. Publication

This edition first published 2009, © 2009 by M. Cruickshank and A. Shetty

Blackwell Publishing was acquired by John Wiley & Sons in February 2007. Blackwell's publishing program has been merged with Wiley's global Scientific, Technical and Medical business to form Wiley-Blackwell.

Registered office: John Wiley & Sons Ltd, The Atrium, Southern Gate, Chichester, West Sussex, PO19 8SQ, UK

Editorial offices: 9600 Garsington Road, Oxford, OX4 2DQ, UK
The Atrium, Southern Gate, Chichester, West Sussex, PO19 8SQ, UK
111 River Street, Hoboken, NJ 07030-5774, USA

For details of our global editorial offices, for customer services and for information about how to apply for permission to reuse the copyright material in this book please see our website at www.wiley.com/wiley-blackwell

Library of Congress Cataloging-in-Publication Data

Cruickshank, Maggie.
    Obstetrics and gynaecology / Maggie Cruickshank, Ashalatha Shetty.
        p.   ;cm. – (Clinical cases uncovered)
    Includes bibliographical references and indexes.
    ISBN 978-1-4051-8671-1
    1. Obstetrics–Case studies.   2. Gynecology–Case studies.   I. Shetty,
Ashalatha.   II. Title.   III. Series: Clinical cases uncovered.
    [DNLM: 1. Pregnancy Complications–diagnosis–Case Reports.   2. Diagnosis,
Differential–Case Reports.   3. Female Urogenital Diseases–diagnosis–Case
Reports.   4. Female Urogenital Diseases–therapy–Case Reports.   5. Pregnancy
Complications–therapy–Case Reports. WQ 240 C955o 2009]
    RG106.C78 2009
    618–dc22

                                                                    2009009649

ISBN: 978-1-4051-8671-1

A catalogue record for this book is available from the British Library.

Set in 9 on 12 pt Minion by SNP Best-set Typesetter Ltd., Hong Kong
Printed and bound in Singapore

1   2009

Contents

Obstetrics

(**Part 3**)   **Self-assessment, 172**

Colour plate section can be found facing p. 84

Preface

For many obstetricians and gynaecologists, the attraction to women's health has been the diversity of our speciality. Obstetrics and gynaecology provides a combination of delivering medical and surgical aspects of care to a range of patients, from the fit and healthy young woman requiring advice or support with health promotion, to the acutely ill woman with severe pre-eclampsia or a ruptured ectopic pregnancy.

The importance of sound scientific knowledge to improve care was highlighted by William Smellie, the 'Father of British Obstetrics' in the 18th century; 'Those who intend to practise Midwifery, ought first of all to make themselves masters of anatomy, and acquire a competent knowledge in surgery and physic; because of their connection with the obstetric art, if not always, at least in many cases' (*A Treatise on the Theory and Practice of Midwifery*. William Smellie 1752).

Obstetrics, gynaecology and sexual health are frequently based on normal physiology incorporating elements of screening, health advice and information alongside an ethical dimension to obstetric and gynaecological practice.

The cases presented in *Obstetrics and Gynaecology: Clinical Cases Uncovered* allow the undergraduate or junior trainee to consider this holistic approach to care which may be lost in a topic- or symptom-based approach. The initial chapters outline the basic underlying science and approach to the patient before embarking on patient-centred cases. The cases have been developed to cover the breadth of women's health and to include commonly encountered clinical scenarios in the clinic or on the ward. They allow the reader to work logically through from the initial consultation, through the rationale for investigations and management plan and key points to consider. Whilst the cases in this book are entirely fictional, they are all based on important or everyday presentations with support and references to essential national guidelines.

Maggie Cruickshank
Ashalatha Shetty

Acknowledgements

We are grateful to many contributors to this book:

Gynaecology

Chris Bain
MD, MRCOG
Consultant Obstetrician and Gynaecologist
Aberdeen Royal Infirmary and Aberdeen Maternity
  Hospital
Cases 5 and 11

Susie Logan
MD (comm), MRCOG, MFSRH
Consultant in Sexual and Reproductive Healthcare
NHS Grampian
Cases 8 and 9

Vanessa Harry
MRCOG
Specialist Registrar, Obstetrics and Gynaecology
Aberdeen Royal Infirmary and Aberdeen Maternity
  Hospital
Cases 2 and 4

Abha Maheshwari
MRCOG
Subspeciality Trainee in Reproductive Medicine
Aberdeen Royal Infirmary and Aberdeen Maternity
  Hospital
Cases 1 and 7

Louise Smart
MD, FRCPath
Consultant Cytopathologist
NHS Grampian
Case 10

Obstetrics

Priya Madhuvrata
MRCOG
Senior Registrar in Obstetrics and Gynaecology
Aberdeen Royal Infirmary and Aberdeen Maternity
  Hospital
Cases 15, 21, 23 and 25

Tara Fairley
MRCOG
Senior Registrar in Obstetrics and Gynaecology
Aberdeen Royal Infirmary and Aberdeen Maternity
  Hospital
Cases 14, 16, 20 and 22

Manisha Mathur
MRCOG
Senior Registrar in Obstetrics and Gynaecology
Aberdeen Royal Infirmary and Aberdeen Maternity
  Hospital
Cases 18, 19, 24 and 26

We would also like to thank Heather Munro for her
invaluable support and effort with typing, collation and
proof reading.

How to use this book

Clinical Cases Uncovered (CCU) books are carefully designed to help supplement your clinical experience and assist with refreshing your memory when revising. Each book is divided into three sections: Part 1, Basics; Part 2, Cases; and Part 3, Self-Assessment.

Part 1 gives a quick reminder of the basic science, history and examination, and key diagnoses in the area. Part 2 contains many of the clinical presentations you would expect to see on the wards or crop up in exams, with questions and answers leading you through each case. New information, such as test results, is revealed as events unfold and each case concludes with a handy case summary explaining the key points. Part 3 allows you to test your learning with several question styles (MCQs, EMQs and SAQs), each with a strong clinical focus.

Whether reading individually or working as part of a group, we hope you will enjoy using your CCU book. If you have any recommendations on how we could improve the series, please do let us know by contacting us at: medstudentuk@oxon.blackwellpublishing.com.

Disclaimer

CCU patients are designed to reflect real life, with their own reports of symptoms and concerns. Please note that all names used are entirely fictitious and any similarity to patients, alive or dead, is coincidental.

List of abbreviations

ABC	airway, breathing, circulation		HAART	highly active antiretroviral therapy
ACE	angiotensin converting enzyme		HBV	hepatitis B virus
AFP	alpha-fetoprotein		HCG	human chorionic gonadotrophin
APH	antepartum haemorrhage		HELLP	(syndrome of) haemolytic anaemia,
ART	antiretroviral therapy			elevated liver enzymes and low platelet
βHCG	β human chorionic gonadotrophin			count
BMD	bone mineral density		HG	hyperemesis gravidarum
BMI	body mass index		HPV	human papillomavirus
BNA	borderline nuclear abnormalities		HRT	hormone replacement therapy
BP	blood pressure		HSV	herpes simplex virus
BV	bacterial vaginosis		HVS	high vaginal swab
CIN	cervical intraepithelial neoplasia		IDDM	insulin-dependent diabetes mellitus
COC	combined oral contraception		Ig	immunoglobulin
CRP	C-reactive protein		IMB	intermenstrual bleeding
CT	computed tomography		IUD	intrauterine device
CTG	cardiotocography/cardiotocogram		IUGR	intrauterine growth restriction
CVD	cardiovascular disease		IUS	intrauterine system
CVS	chorionic villus sampling		IVF	*in vitro* fertilization
DIC	disseminated intravascular coagulopathy		LARC	long-acting reversible contraception
DLA	daily living activity		LAVH	laparoscopic-assisted vaginal hysterectomy
DMPA	depo-medroxyprogesterone acetate		LEI	liver enzyme inducer
DUB	dysfunctional uterine bleeding		LFT	liver function test
EB	endometrial biopsy		LH	luteinizing hormone
EC	emergency contraception		LLETZ	large loop excision of transformation zone
ECG	electrocardiography/electrocardiogram		LMP	last menstrual period
ECV	external cephalic version		LNG-IUS	levonorgestrel-releasing intrauterine
EDD	expected date of delivery			system
ERCS	elective repeat caesarean section		MAP	mean arterial pressure
EUA	examination under anaesthesia		MEA	microwave endometrial ablation
FBC	full blood count		MRI	magnetic resonance imaging
FIGO	International Federation of Gynaecology		MSSU	mid-stream specimen of urine
	and Obstetrics		NAAT	nucleic acid amplification test
FSH	follicle stimulating hormone		NFP	natural family planning
FVU	first void urine		NICE	National Institute for Clinical Excellence
GDM	gestational diabetes mellitus		NNRTI	non-nucleoside reverse transcriptase
GFR	glomerular filtration rate			inhibitor
GMC	General Medical Council		NRTI	nucleoside reverse transcriptase inhibitor
GnRH	gonadotrophin releasing hormone		NSAID	non-steroidal anti-inflammatory drug
GUM	genitourinary medicine		NT	nuchal translucency

NTD	neural tube defect
OGTT	oral glucose tolerance test
OSCE	objective structured clinical examination
PAPP-A	pregnancy-associated plasma protein A
PCA	patient-controlled opioid analgesia
PCB	postcoital bleeding
PCOS	polycystic ovarian syndrome
PI	protease inhibitor
PID	pelvic inflammatory disease
PLCS	prelabour caesarean section
PMB	postmenopausal bleeding
POI	progesterone only implant
POP	progesterone only pill
PPH	postpartum haemorrhage
PPROM	preterm premature rupture of membranes
PRL	prolactin
PROM	premature rupture of membranes
PV	per vaginum
RCOG	Royal College of Obsteticians and Gynaecologists
RhD	rhesus D
RMI	Risk of Malignancy Index
SCJ	squamocolumnar junction
SFH	symphysiofundal height

SOLVS	self-obtained low vaginal swab
START	short-term antiretroviral therapy
STI	sexually transmitted infection
TAH/BSO	total abdominal hysterectomy and bilateral salpingo-oopherectomy
TED	thromboembolic disease
TENS	transcutaneous electrical nerve stimulation
TFT	thyroid function test
TPN	total parenteral nutrition
TRAP	twin reversed arterial perfusion
TSH	thyroid stimulating hormone
TTTS	twin–twin transfusion syndrome
TV US	transvaginal ultrasound
TZ	transformation zone
U&E	urea and electrolytes
uE3	unconjugated estriol
UTI	urinary tract infection
VBAC	vaginal birth after caesarean section
VIN	vulval intraepithelial neoplasia
VTE	venous thromboembolism
VVC	vulvovaginal candiasis
ZDV	ziduvidine

Basic science: gynaecology

The female reproductive tract can be divided into the lower and the upper genital tracts from a functional and clinical viewpoint.

Lower genital tract

The lower genital tract comprises the vulva, vagina and cervix.

The vulva
Development

In early embryonic development there is a common indifferent stage when the external genitalia of both sexes comprises:

- Two genital swellings
- Two genital folds
- A midline anterior genital tubercle

In the absence of fetal testosterone, these develop in the female into:

- Labia majora
- Labia minora
- Clitoris

During puberty, there is an increase in the size of the labia majora and pubis by the accumulation of fat, and pubic hair develops prior to menarche. Low oestrogen levels after the menopause result in atrophic changes with loss of fat and pubic hair and sometimes narrowing of the introitus.

Anatomy

The vulva has a rich blood supply from the internal pudendal artery and other branches of the internal iliac artery, and the external pudendal artery which arises from the femoral artery (Fig. A).

Obstetrics and Gynaecology: Clinical Cases Uncovered.
By M. Cruickshank and A. Shetty. Published 2009 by Blackwell Publishing. ISBN 978-1-4051-8671-1.

The lymphatics drain to the inguinal and superficial femoral lymph nodes. The pudendal nerves arise from S2, 3 and 4.

The vagina
Development

The upper vagina develops from the paramesonephric duct and the lower vagina forms by canalization of the solid sinovaginal valves. The introitus and the hymen develop from the urogenital sinus. The complete canalization of the vagina does not occur until 6–7 months *in utero*.

Anatomy

The vagina is lined by stratified squamous epithelium. This epithelium is rich in glycogen; a substrate used by the normal commensal lactobacillus. The breakdown of glycogen to lactic acid produces an acidic vaginal pH. This has a protective role in maintaining normal vaginal flora and preventing an overgrowth of pathogenic organisms.

Secretions from the cervical, paraurethral and Bartholin's glands and some vaginal transudate form physiological vaginal discharge. Before puberty and after the menopause low oestrogen levels are associated with low levels of glycogen and thinning of the vaginal mucosa.

The blood supply derives from the vaginal artery branch of the internal iliac artery.

The lymphatic drainage from the lower third of the vagina is the same as the vulva but the upper two-thirds drain to the internal iliac, obturator and external iliac nodes.

The cervix
Development

The cervix and the uterus develop from the fusion of the paramesonephric ducts with absorption of the central septum to form a single cavity. The cervix projects into the vaginal vault and the ectocervical portion is covered

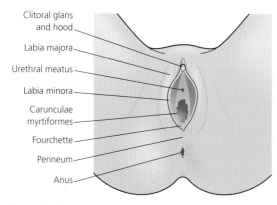

Clitoral glans and hood
Labia majora
Urethral meatus
Labia minora
Carunculae myrtiformes
Fourchette
Perineum
Anus

Figure A Vulval anatomy.

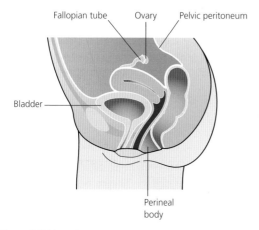

Fallopian tube   Ovary   Pelvic peritoneum

Bladder

Perineal body

Figure B Pelvic anatomy.

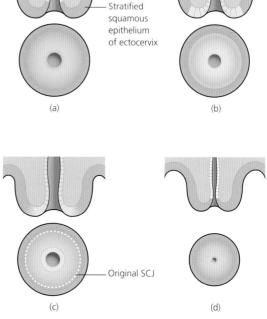

Stratified squamous epithelium of ectocervix

(a)   (b)

Original SCJ

(c)   (d)

Figure C Cervical epithelium and the influence of oestrogen. (a) Prepuberty. Original squamocolumnar junction (SCJ) seen at external cervical os. (b) At puberty, the SCJ is seen out on the surface of the ectocervix exposing the columnar epithelium (ectopy). (c) The exposed columnar epithelium undergoes metaplasia. (d) Low oestrogen levels shrink the cervix and the SCJ retracts into the endocervical canal after the menopause.

with the same stratified squamous epithelium as the vagina. By contrast, the endocervical canal has a single layer of columnar epithelium and contains numerous mucus glands. The two types of epithelium meet at the original squamocolumnar junction (SCJ) and *in utero*, under the effect of maternal oestrogens, this lies on the surface of the ectocervix. The site of the SCJ changes after birth and throughout reproductive life.

The transformation zone of the cervix

Low oestrogen levels in childhood result in the SCJ retracting into the endocervical canal. During puberty, increasing oestrogen levels increases the size of the cervix with eversion of the anterior and posterior lips of the cervix. This exposes the columnar epithelium which appears redder and rougher than the smooth pale squamous epithelium. This is a physiological change called

an ectopy or ectropion. The acidic pH of the vagina promotes active metaplasia of columnar to squamous epithelium. As a result, the original SCJ junction lies out on the ectocervix and the area between this and the new SCJ is known as the transformation zone (TZ). The endocervix contains many mucous glands and gland openings can still be seen within the TZ. Cervical mucus produces most of the vaginal secretions.

The TZ is the area where precancerous and cancerous changes are most likely to be identified (see Case 10) and this is the area of the cervix that needs to be sampled for cervical screening. After the menopause, reduced oestrogen levels produce shrinkage of the cervix and retraction of the SCJ into the endocervical canal.

The cervix receives its blood supply from ascending branches from the vaginal artery and descending branches from the uterine artery.

The lymphatics drain to the internal and external iliac and the obturator fossa nodes.

Upper genital tract

The upper genital tract comprises the uterus, fallopian tubes and ovaries.

The uterus
Development

While the uterus forms by fusion of the paramesonephric duct, the mesonephric ducts in the female fetus degenerate after the indifferent stage. The upper part of the paramesonephric ducts remain separate and form the fallopian tubes. These enter through the thick muscular walls of the uterus at the cornua and on hysteroscopy the tubal ostia can be seen at either end of the uterine fundus. Inferiorly, the upper end of the endocervical canal is known as the internal os.

Anatomy

The outer surface of the myometrium is covered by peritoneum which runs over the dome of the bladder and posteriorly to cover the pouch of Douglas behind the uterus and upper vagina. Lateral to the body of the uterus, this forms the broad ligament which is simply a fold of peritoneum which has no supportive function.

The uterus receives its blood supply from the uterine artery, a branch of the internal iliac artery. It crosses the ureter and runs a very tortuous course up the side of the uterus. This allows the large increase in size of the uterus during pregnancy.

The lymphatics drain to the internal and external iliac and the obturator fossa nodes.

> **KEY POINT**
>
> It is important to know the anatomical course of the ureter for gynaecological surgery as it passes through the base of the broad ligament and close to the cervix

The endometrium

The inner layer of the uterus is the endometrium. The basal layer of the endometrium remains throughout the menstrual cycle and forms tubular glands which penetrate into the myometrium. The endometrial structure and function is controlled by hormones which vary throughout the menstrual cycle.

- *Following menstruation.* The basal layer is covered by necrotic glandular and stromal tissue with the underlying glands intact.
- *Proliferative phase.* There is rapid repair of the endometrial glands and stromal metaplasia. Initially, the surface epithelium is thin but by mid-cycle it is 3 mm in thickness. The endometrial glands are formed by a single layer of cuboidal cells with a short straight narrow lumen.
- *Following ovulation* (early secretory phase). Increasing oestrogen and progesterone production stimulates secretory activity (the secretory phase of endometrium). The glands lengthen and become tortuous. This prepares the endometrium for implantation should the ovum be fertilized.
- *Later secretory phase.* Progesterone decidualizes the endometrial stroma with increased size of the stromal cells and increased extracellular fluid. If pregnancy does not occur, the endometrium undergoes apoptosis and consequently loss of the functional outer 75% of the endometrium.

The ovary

The ovaries are essential to reproductive function with ovum production and oestrogen and progesterone production under the control of the hypothalamic pituitary axis.

Development

The primitive gonads first appear at 5 weeks' gestation as a gonadal streak in the mesonephric genital ridge. At this indifferent stage, they can develop into ovaries or testicles. These contain coelomic epithelium, mesoderm and primitive germ cells. The primitive germ cells originate in the endoderm and migrate to the primitive gonad to develop into oocytes. The stromal cells develop from the ovarian mesenchyme. The number of oocytes is greatest *in utero* before birth and throughout life many oocytes undergo atresia. The ovum remains in arrested meiosis and this is not completed unless the oocyte is fertilized by a sperm.

The gonads descend from the abdominal cavity into the pelvis in the female, and the scrotum in the male, by a ligament known as the gubernaculum. This embryological remnant is called the round ligament and has no supportive structure in the female.

Anatomy

The ovaries are suspended from the back of the cornua of the uterus by the ovarian ligament and from the broad ligament by the mesovarian, which contains the nerves and vessels, and laterally to the suspensory ligament. In

Table A The menstrual cycle.

Menstrual cycle		Day	Hypothalamus and pituitary	Ovary	Endometrium
Follicular phase	Menstruation Development of the oocyte	1 5	↑ FSH ↓ FSH because of **negative** feedback of increasing oestrogen	Stimulates development of 10–20 primary follicles Follicles mature with increasing production of oestrogen Dominant follicle emerges	Endometrial shedding Endometrial repair Vasoconstriction Endometrial proliferation Growth of glands and stroma
Ovulation	Mid cycle	14	Feedback effect of oestrogen changes to **positive** with peak release of GnRH, LH surge and small peak of FSH	16–24 hours post LH surge, dominant follicle releases ovum	
Luteal phase			FSH inhibited	Luteinization of theca-granulosa cells of dominant follicle	Progesterone production ↑ glandular secretory activity
		22 24	If no pregnancy, falling oestrogen and progesterone levels result in positive feedback and ↑ FSH		Decidualization Degeneration of endometrium
	Menstruation	1			Endometrial shedding

FSH, follicle stimulating hormone; GnRH, gonadotrophin releasing hormone; LH, luteinizing hormone.

the front of the ovary lies the fallopian tube with the fimbrial end close to the ovary.

The blood supply to the ovary comes from the ovarian arteries directly off the aorta below the level of the renal arteries. The right ovarian vein drains into the inferior vena cava and on the left into the left renal vein.

Lymphatic drainage of the ovary follows the course of the blood vessels to the para-aortic lymph nodes.

The ovaries consist of a central vascular medulla and outer denser cortex covered with a single layer of cuboidal cells. The outer cortex contains oocyte follicles at various stages of development. Both the cortex and the medulla contain stroma which provide support and structure to the ovary but also synthesize steroid hormones. The majority of the primordial follicles present at birth undergo atresia and it is the developing follicle that produces circulating oestrogens. Oestrogen is synthesized principally from androstenedione and testosterone to oestradiol by the granulosa cells which line the follicle.

Reproductive physiology
Puberty
Stimulation of ovarian tissue comes from follicle stimulating hormone (FSH) and luteinizing hormones (LH). These are produced from the pituitary gland. FSH is suppressed in the fetus by oestrogens from placental and maternal sources. In childhood, FSH levels are raised as a result of low oestrogen levels. FSH is centrally inhibited by gonadotrophin releasing hormones (GnRH) produced from the hypothalamus. In the 2 years prior to puberty, pulsatile release of FSH starts and increases in frequency until it reaches normal adult levels. This establishes the menstrual cycle.

KEY POINT

In the first years following menarche, cycles can be anovulatory which results in irregular and sometimes heavy and painful periods

Menstrual cycle

Ovarian hormone production is controlled by the pituitary and hypothalamus and the menstrual cycle results if pregnancy is not achieved (Table A).

Menopause

Even before the perimenopause, FSH levels start to increase with altered ovarian response. Periods may become lighter and less frequent or stop abruptly as ovulation ceases. Progesterone production is reduced which affects luteinization. Despite rising FSH levels, ovarian follicles fail to respond to gonadotrophins and oestrogen production falls.

After the menopause, oestrone is found in lower levels and is mainly produced by peripheral conversion of androstenidione in adipose tissue.

Support to the pelvic floor and organs

The pelvic floor is formed by the levator ani muscles which rise in a line running along the lower part of the pubic bone, the internal surface of the pelvic fascia and the ischial spine. They insert into the midline, the wall of the anal canal and the lower part of the coccyx.

The urogenital diaphragm lies below the levator ani and fills the gap between the pubic rami. The urethra and vagina both pass through this diaphragm in the midline.

Another important supporting structure is the perineal body, a condensation of muscle between the lower third of the vagina and the anal canal. Its boundaries are the vaginal fourchette to the anus and, superiorly, the point where the posterior vaginal wall and the rectum meet. Damage may occur following childbirth from tears and care needs to be taken to identify any disruption for repair.

The main supporting structures to the uterus are the uterosacral ligaments and the transverse cervical ligaments. The uterosacral ligaments are dense fibrous cords running from the posterior wall of the cervix and the vaginal vault to the sacrum and can be clearly seen at laparoscopy. The transverse cervical ligaments insert at the level of the cervix and vaginal vault and spread out laterally to the pelvic side wall. These lie under the base of the broad ligament and cannot be seen unless the pelvic side wall is opened. Both these pairs of ligaments transmit sympathetic and parasympathetic nerve supply to the pelvic organs.

Basic science: obstetrics

PART 1: BASICS

Pregnancy involves a number of changes to the maternal physiology, anatomy and hormonal milieu, to allow for optimal growth and development of the fetus, protect the mother through the processes of pregnancy and birth, and also to allow for nurturing of the newborn baby. Some of these normal physiological changes may result in maternal symptoms and changes in the results of clinical investigations which may, in the non-pregnant state, be associated with disease, and could therefore confuse clinical assessment.

The placenta

Implantation of the embryo into the endometrium occurs 8–10 days after fertilization. The surface trophoblastic cells of the blastocyst differentiate into the cytotrophoblast and the syntiotrophoblast which proliferate and penetrate the uterine decidua and go on to form the placenta. The placenta is an efficient interface between the fetal vascular surface and that of the mother and allows the fetus to obtain nutrients, exchange gases and eliminate its waste products.

The placenta is also a major endocrine organ. It synthesizes and secretes steroid hormones – progestogens and oestrogens – and a number of other hormones including human chorionic gonadotrophin, relaxin and placental lactogen, all of which have profound effects on both fetal and maternal physiology.

Human chorionic gonadotrophin

This is one of the earliest hormones synthesized by the chorion. It maintains the corpus luteum in the ovary, which secretes progesterone and oestrogen, both of which are essential for maintenance of the pregnancy,

until the placenta takes over the production of these hormones (by about 8 weeks' gestation).

Progesterone

This is one of the major hormones that helps maintain the pregnancy. It appears to decrease the maternal immune response to allow for the acceptance of the pregnancy, and decreases contractility of the uterine smooth muscle allowing it to hold the pregnancy until labour and delivery. A drop in progesterone levels possibly facilitates the onset of labour.

Its relaxing effects on the smooth muscle are also seen on the ureters, oesophageal sphincter and the intestines. These may result in clinical symptoms of reflux, heartburn, delayed gastric emptying, constipation and ureteric dilatation which may contribute to the increase in urinary tract infection and/or pylonephrites in pregnancy.

Oestrogen (oestriol, oestradiol and oestrone)

While the placenta is the main source of oestrogen, it requires certain enzymes that are produced by the fetus to complete its synthesis. Oestrogen promotes the growth of uterine muscle to allow it to adapt to the growing pregnancy. Changes in the breast to allow milk production by increasing duct and alveolar development and to allow feeding by increasing the size and mobility of the nipple are also promoted by oestrogen. It increases protein synthesis, and has effects on blood volume and coagulation. It causes changes in the cervix including softening to prepare it for labour.

Relaxin

Relaxin facilitates the birth process by causing a softening of the cervix and the ligaments of pubic symphysis, by simultaneously reducing collagen production and increasing collagen breakdown. The loosening of the ligaments of the symphysis pubis can result in maternal discomfort and symphysis pubis diasthesis, especially in the later stages of pregnancy.

Obstetrics and Gynaecology: Clinical Cases Uncovered. By M. Cruickshank and A. Shetty. Published 2009 by Blackwell Publishing. ISBN 978-1-4051-8671-1.

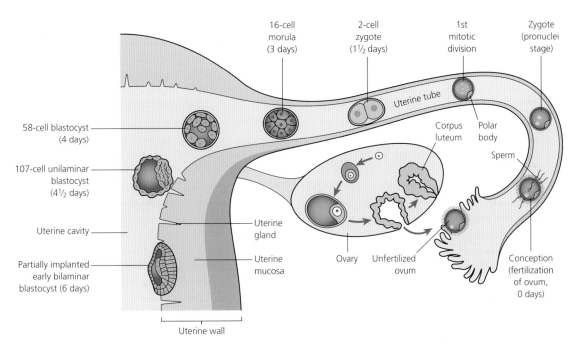

Figure D Ovulation to blastocyst formation.

Transfer across the placenta

Feto-maternal exchange across the placenta may be *passive* (by simple diffusion, e.g. for water, oxygen, carbon dioxide, urea), *facilitated* by a carrier molecule (e.g. for glucose), *active* by enzymatic action (e.g. amnio acids, free fatty acids, water-soluble vitamins) or by *pinocytosis* (e.g. immunoglobulin G [IgG] antibodies, lipoproteins).

Most medications or drugs pass through the placenta as do nicotine, alcohol and illegal substances such as cocaine and heroin. This is particularly important in the first trimester for drugs that may be teratogenic, e.g. angiotensin converting enzyme (ACE) inhibitors, but may also be of relevance later on in pregnancy, for example when there is neonatal withdrawal from opiates.

The embryo and fetus

In humans, the embryonic period begins at fertilization (2 weeks' gestation or about 2 weeks after the last menstrual period in a 28-day cycle) and continues until the end of the eighth week of development (10 weeks' gestation).

Following fertilization once the zygote is formed, it travels down the fallopian tube, dividing several times as it does so, to form a ball of cells called a morula. Further cellular division is accompanied by the formation of a small cavity between the cells, resulting in a blastocyst. The blastocyst reaches the uterine cavity at approximately the fifth day after fertilization. Lysis of the zona pellucida, the glycoprotein shell around the blastocyst, occurs, so that it can come into contact with and become embedded in the uterine endometrium (implantation).

In most successful pregnancies, the blastocyst implants 8–10 days after ovulation. The inner cell mass forms the embryo, while the outer cell layers form the membranes and placenta. Together, the embryo and its membranes are referred to as a conceptus, or the 'products of conception'.

At this stage, there is rapid growth of the embryo, and by the end of the embryonic period (10 weeks' gestation or eighth week of development) the beginnings of all essential structures are in place and the embryo's main external features begin to take form. This process is called differentiation, and it results in the varied cell types (such as blood, kidney and nerve cells). A miscarriage or birth defects may occur if there are genetic abnormalities in the developing embryo, or toxic exposures, for example, to infections (e.g. rubella and cytomegalovirus), alcohol, certain drugs or nutritional deficiencies (e.g. folate, which might result in open neural tube defects). In the vast majority of early miscarriages, however, it is difficult to determine the causative factor.

The fetal period extends from 10 weeks' gestation to birth and is characterized by growth and elaboration of the structures and organ systems. Genitals are well differentiated by 12 weeks' gestation, and by 19–20 weeks nails appear on toes and fingers and the mother is usually able to feel 'quickening' – small fetal movements (although in parous women, quickening may be felt much earlier than at 20 weeks).

Some of the factors affecting fetal size and growth *in utero* include race, ethnicity, size (body mass index [BMI]), parity, age of the mother (e.g. teenage mothers may have small babies), smoking, alcohol and drug misuse, pre-eclampsia, recurrent antepartum haemorrhages, diabetes (usually causes large babies, but may result in growth restricted babies with severe disease), multiple gestation, maternal infections and fetal congenital abnormalities.

Adaptation of the fetus to extrauterine life

The circulatory system of a human fetus works differently from that of adults, mainly because the lungs are not in use: the fetus obtains oxygen and nutrients from the mother through the placenta. Blood from the placenta is carried to the fetus by the umbilical vein. About half of this enters the fetal ductus venosus and is carried to the inferior vena cava, while the other half enters the liver. The branch of the umbilical vein that supplies the right lobe of the liver first joins with the portal vein. The blood then moves to the right atrium of the heart, from where most of it flows through the foramen ovale (opening between the right and left atrium) directly into the left atrium, thus bypassing pulmonary circulation. The continuation of this blood flow is then into the left ventricle, from where it is pumped through the aorta into the body. Some of the blood moves from the aorta through the internal iliac arteries to the umbilical arteries, and re-enters the placenta, where carbon dioxide and other waste products from the fetus are taken up by the mother's circulation.

Some of the blood entering the right atrium does not pass directly to the left atrium through the foramen ovale, but enters the right ventricle and is pumped into the pulmonary artery. In the fetus, there is a special connection between the pulmonary artery and the aorta, the ductus arteriosus, which directs most of this blood away from the lungs.

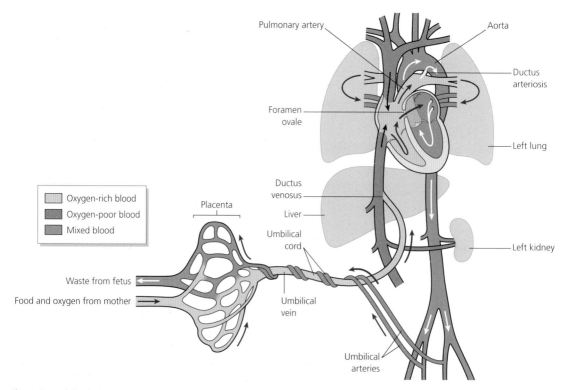

Figure E Fetal circulation.

Once the baby is born and the first breath is taken, the circulatory and respiratory systems change dramatically. The pulmonary resistance is reduced, and more blood moves from the right atrium to the right ventricle and into the pulmonary arteries, and less flows through the foramen ovale to the left atrium. The blood from the lungs travels through the pulmonary veins to the left atrium, increasing the pressure there. The decreased right atrial pressure and the increased left atrial pressure results in the closure of the foramen ovale, which now becomes the fossa ovalis. This completes the separation of the circulatory system into two halves, the left and the right.

The ductus arteriosus normally closes off within 1–2 days of birth, leaving behind the ligamentum arteriosum. The umbilical vein and the ductus venosus close within 2–5 days after birth, leaving behind the ligamentum teres and the ligamentum venosus of the liver, respectively.

Changes in the pregnant mother

Maternal changes start from very early on in the first trimester of the pregnancy. Nearly all systems are affected.

Cardiac system

Stroke volume and heart rate both increase resulting in cardiac output increasing by about 40% (from 4 to 6 L/min). The pulse rate may increase by 10–15 beats/minute. The increased flow across the heart valves results in an increase in physiological flow murmurs heard on auscultation.

There is a decrease in peripheral vascular resistance, resulting in a fall in blood pressure of about 10 mmHg in mean arterial pressure (MAP) in the first and second trimesters. The blood pressure tends to rise again after about 24 weeks' gestation.

The gravid uterus, especially in the later stages of pregnancy, can occlude the inferior vena cava when the mother lies flat on her back, and cause decreased return of blood to the heart, hypotension and reduced fetal flow (supine hypotension). This is why pregnant mothers are advised not to lie flat on their backs, and labour, delivery and anaesthesia are managed with the mother propped up or with a wedge that tilts her back.

Respiratory system

There is increased oxygen requirement in pregnancy, which results in hyperventilation and deep breathing. Ventilation is increased by 40% through an increase in tidal volume (from 500 to 700 mL) rather than in the respiratory rate. CO_2 levels in pregnancy are lower than in the non-pregnant state; this helps the gradient between fetus and mother and favours transfer of CO_2 from fetus to mother across the placenta. Mothers may feel dyspnoeic; this may partly be because of the splinting of the diaphragm by the gravid uterus.

Body temperature

Progesterone is thought to be responsible for the rise in body temperature of 0.5–1.0°C during pregnancy. An increased metabolic rate and peripheral vasodilatation also result in a warm skin and may cause palmar erythema.

Blood and plasma volume

Blood volume increases by approximately 1200 mL (40%), while red cell mass increases by 250–400 mL (about 25%). This results in a relative haemodilution and anaemia, with a drop in haematocrit and haemoglobin levels.

There is increased blood flow to a number of systems including the uterus, skin and the kidneys. There is an increase in the glomerular filtration rate (GFR) from 140 to 170 mL/minute. This results in lower serum urea and creatinine levels. This needs to be borne in mind when interpreting blood results in pregnancy, as the normal range quoted for the non-pregnant state may not be relevant, and an abnormal result may be missed.

There is an increase in extravascular fluid because of lower plasma colloid osmotic pressure (albumin levels are lower in pregnancy), and this contributes to the peripheral odema that may be seen with normal pregnancy. Symptoms of carpel tunnel syndrome of tingling of the fingers may be caused by compression of the median nerve under the flexor retinaculum because of increased extracellular fluid.

The blood may show a mild leucocytosis in pregnancy ($9–11 \times 10^9$/L compared to $4–11 \times 10^9$/L) and an increase in erythrocyte sedimentation rate. Serum iron is lower and iron requirements are increased because of demands from the fetus, red cell increase and blood loss at delivery. There is no consensus as to whether routine iron supplementation is indicated in pregnancy but evidence suggests that a higher iron level following supplementation does not improve maternal or neonatal outcomes. Iron supplementation is advised at haemoglobin levels below 10.5 gm/dL.

Metabolic changes

Metabolic rate is increased to accommodate increased energy demands from the fetus and for the maternal changes. Pregnancy is also a diabetogenic state. Glucose levels are increased as placental hormones are insulin antagonists and there is an increased insulin resistance in pregnancy. If sufficient insulin cannot be produced to counter this resistance, gestational diabetes may occur. This physiological change also explains why insulin requirements in known insulin-dependent diabetic mothers increases during pregnancy.

Coagulation profile

Pregnancy is a hypercoagulable state. This is a protective mechanism for the mother to be able to minimize blood loss after delivery of the placenta. There is an increase in fibrinogen, factor VIII and von Willebrand factor, and a decrease in anticoagulants such as antithrombin III. There is also an increase in fibrinolytic activity.

While this hypercoagulable state is protective against bleeding, it results in an increased risk of thrombosis during pregnancy, especially when there are other risk factors present (e.g. increasing age, smoking, high BMI, operative delivery, prolonged immobilization).

Maternal weight gain

This is around 11–12 kg through the pregnancy. Much of this increase is caused by the extravascular retention of fluid (approximately 8.5 L), increase in blood volume, growth of the uterus, breasts and body fat. The fetus (around 3.5 kg), placenta and liquor (about 0.7–0.8 kg each) account for about 4.5–5 kg of the weight gain.

Other changes

There may be thyroid enlargement and a mild goitre in pregnancy. As there is increased urinary excretion of iodine and some uptake of iodothyronines by the fetus, there is a relative iodine deficiency in the mother. This results in a compensatory thyroid hypertrophy in order to maintain normal iodide concentrations. Especially in early pregnancy, blood results may mimic a hyperthyroid state with low thyroid stimulating hormone (TSH), but free T_3 and T_4 remain within the normal range. In mothers with a known history of hypothyroidism, thyroid requirements may increase in pregnancy.

Renal changes include anatomical ones (dilatation of renal pelvis and ureters) brought about by both the effects of progesterone and pressure effects from the growing gravid uterus to some extent. Renal function tests change in pregnancy. Glycosuria may occur in the presence of normal plasma glucose levels, because of an increase in the GFR and a change in tubular reabsorption of glucose.

The uterus undergoes both hypertrophy and hyperplasia, and increases from a non-pregnant weight of 0.3–0.4 kg to 1–1.3 kg at term. Uterine blood flow increases from 50 to 500 mL/minute.

The narrow isthmus of the uterus between the body of the uterus and the cervix becomes increasing stretched

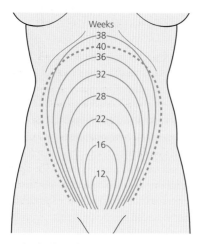

Figure F Uterine height with increasing gestation.

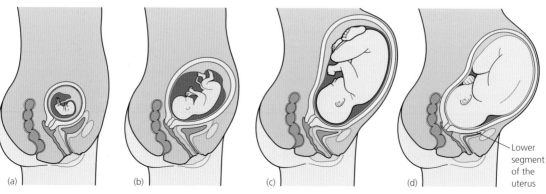

Figure G Progressive enlargement of the lower segment of the uterus with increasing gestation (a)–(d).

PART 1: BASICS

and thinned out as the pregnancy progresses, to become the well-formed lower segment at term. This is the preferred site for the uterine incision at caesarean section, because of its relative avascularity, quiescence, better healing and lower risk of scar rupture in a subsequent pregnancy than an upper segment incision. The lower segment does not contract during labour.

As labour progresses, the cervix dilates and effaces almost completely into the lower segment. When the placenta is low lying and implanted on the lower segment, there is an increased risk of postpartum haemorrhage as the lower segment does not contract effectively after delivery of the placenta.

As pregnancy progresses, the collagen concentration in the cervix decreases and there is accumulation of glycosaminoglycans and water. This results in increasing 'ripening' of the cervix in preparation for labour.

Labour

Labour is the process whereby the fetus is delivered from the mother; it involves regular uterine activity causing progressive cervical dilatation and effacement followed by expulsion of the fetus.

There are no conclusive theories to explain the onset of labour. A change in the levels of and ratio between concentrations of oestrogen and progesterone has been suggested, possibly following a fetal trigger in the form of secretion of adrenal corticosteroids when it is mature and ready to be delivered. Prostaglandin concentrations have been shown to increase prelabour and they are known to promote cervical ripening and uterine contractility. Oxytocin receptors in the uterus also increase towards term and oxytocin from the posterior pituitary is known to be a potent stimulator of uterine contractions.

The diagnosis of active labour is not always easy and includes the presence of regular painful contractions with increasing effacement and dilatation (usually at least 3–4 cm) of the cervix. There may be a 'show' (bloodstained mucosal discharge) associated with the cervical changes. The first stage of labour is defined as the period from the start of active labour until full (10 cm) cervical dilatation.

The second stage includes the time until delivery of the fetus after full cervical dilatation ('active' second stage is when the mother is actively pushing with uterine contractions, while 'passive' second stage is when time is allowed for the head to descend lower into the pelvis by uterine contractions alone without maternal effort).

The third stage includes the time from delivery of the fetus to the delivery of the placenta. The signs of placental separation include lengthening of the cord, a gush of blood vaginally and sustained contraction of the uterus.

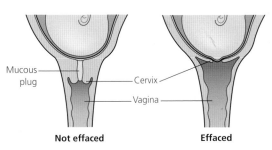

Figure H Cerival changes in labour.

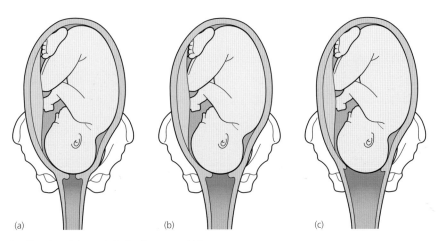

Figure I Progessive dilatation of the cervix in the first stage of labour.

Puerperium is the period following delivery which lasts about 6–8 weeks, when the body returns to its prepregnant state. While much of the physiological and anatomical change is reversed, some changes are lasting (e.g. the presence of stria gravidarum). It is important to remember that some of the maternal changes of pregnancy (e.g. the hypercoagulable state) remain for some time after delivery and therefore the risks (e.g. of thrombosis) remain too.

Approach to the patient

The gynaecological patient

Most diagnoses are made from the patient's history and examination so this should be taken carefully and systematically. At the start of the consultation always introduce yourself, giving your name and position, and ask for consent whenever examining a patient. This is particularly important if you are going to perform a pelvic examination (Box A).

The general structure of a gynaecology consultation follows that of any other system but there are additional history sections for relevant important information such as a menstrual history and past obstetric history. This is particularly important if the patient is currently pregnant but will contribute to any gynaecological history.

Presenting complaint

The consultation starts with an open question to determine the presenting complaint. Remember that much of obstetric and gynaecological practice relates to normality and promoting good reproductive health. The patient may be referred for an opinion despite feeling perfectly well and may not have a complaint as such. The patient's perception of a problem may be quite different from the details in the referral letter and it is best to start with open questions to invite the patient to explain in her own words what has been happening.

Menstrual history

It is worthwhile at the start to check on the date of the patient's last menstrual period (LMP).
• The menstrual cycle is represented by the letter κ = numerator/denominator
• The numerator is the total number of days that she bleeds for

Obstetrics and Gynaecology: Clinical Cases Uncovered.
By M. Cruickshank and A. Shetty. Published 2009 by Blackwell Publishing. ISBN 978-1-4051-8671-1.

• The denominator is the length of the menstrual cycle from the first day of one period to the first day of her next period
• If the patient does not have a regular cycle, this should be expressed as a range from the minimum length of the cycle to the maximum length of the cycle
• κ = 5/28 describes a woman who bleeds for 5 days with a regular 28-day cycle

Abnormal vaginal bleeding

It is usual to ask about the age of the first menstruation (menarche). You need to ask about intermenstrual bleeding (IMB) and postcoital bleeding (PCB) which is provoked by intercourse. If the patient is postmenopausal, ask about the date of her last normal period and if she has experienced any vaginal bleeding since then. Postmenopausal bleeding (PMB) is bleeding more than 1 year after the last normal period (Table B).

Heavy menstrual bleeding

If the patient complains of heavy periods, there are a number of ways in which the severity is assessed but the most important aspect is the effect on patient's quality of life such as whether it disrupts her normal activities.

Clots

Normal menstrual blood does not clot because of the local release of prostaglandins. The formation of clots suggests that the blood loss overwhelms this natural system. It is important to assess the size of the clots. As clots often form in the vagina, they tend to be like pieces of liver.

Sanitary protection

It is useful to ask about:
• Sanitary protection, including the strength of absorbency of sanitary pads or tampons
• Frequency of changing pads or tampons

Box A General Medical Council (GMC) guidelines on intimate examination

1 Intimate examinations

Whenever you are examining a patient you should be sensitive as to what they may perceive as intimate. This is likely to include examinations of breast, genitalia and rectum but could also include any examination where it is necessary to touch or even be close to the patient

2 Chaperones

- Whenever possible you should offer the patient an impartial observer (a chaperone). This applies whether or not you are the same gender as the patient
- A chaperone does not have to be medically qualified but should be:
  - respectful of the patient's dignity and confidentiality
  - prepared to reassure the patient
  - familiar with the procedures involved in a routine intimate examination
  - be prepared to raise concerns about a doctor
- If either you or the patient does not wish the examination to proceed without a chaperone present you may offer to delay the examination if this is compatible with the patient's best interest
- You should record any discussion about chaperones and its outcome. If a chaperone is present you should record their identity. If the patient does not want a chaperone you should record that the offer was made and declined

3 Communication in relation to intimate examinations

Before conducting an intimate examination you should:

- Explain to the patient the purpose of the examination and give her an opportunity to ask questions
- Explain what the examination will involve so the patient has a clear idea of what to expect
- Obtain the patient's permission before the examination
- Give the patient privacy to undress and dress
- Keep the patient covered as much as possible to maintain dignity

During the examination you should:

- Explain what you are going to do beforehand
- Discontinue the examination if the patient asks you to
- Keep discussion relevant
- Avoid unnecessary personal comments

When examining anaesthetized patients:

- You must obtain consent for the examination prior to anaesthetic
- The supervisor of students needs to ensure that valid consent has been obtained before allowing students to conduct an intimate examination under anaesthesia

---

Term	Definition
Menarche	Age at first menstruation
Menopause	Date of last normal period
Amenorrhoea	No menstrual bleeding
Oligomenorrhoea	Infrequent menstruation
Menorrhagia	Heavy regular menstrual bleeding
Metromenorrhagia	Heavy irregular menstrual bleeding
Intermenstrual bleeding (IMB)	Bleeding in between periods
Postcoital bleeding (PCB)	Bleeding after penetrative sex
Postmenopausal bleeding (PMB)	Bleeding after the menopause
Dysmenorrhoea	Pain associated with menstruation
κ (cycle) = N/D	= no of days of bleeding/total length of menstrual cycle
Dyspareunia	Pain associated with penetrative sex

Table B Definitions of gynaecological terms.

- Double protection (wearing a pad in addition to a tampon)
- Use of towels or other covers to protect the bed during the night

Flooding

Flooding means the menstrual loss is heavy enough to soak through outer clothes but some staining of underwear is considered normal.

Contraception

As part of the menstrual history you should also ask about her method of contraception and any problems associated with this.

Cervical smears

In the UK, all women are called on a regular basis for cervical screening but it is worth checking that they have complied with screening and have a smear result within their last screening round. Remember that the eligible age group for screening varies in different screening programmes.

Pain

To assist your diagnosis, you need to establish if pelvic pain is cyclical or non-cyclical and if cyclical, in which part in the menstrual cycle pain occurs. You also need to enquire about dysparunia (pain during sexual intercourse). This may be superficial (on penetration) or deep (within the pelvis). Further information on site, radiation, character, aggravating and relieving factors follows the same format as other systems.

Past obstetric history

A more detailed past obstetric history would be required for an obstetric patient. You still require a past obstetric history from gynaecology patients; it is normal to note the number of previous pregnancies, the gestation reached and the outcome for the pregnancy. For patients with urinary or prolapse symptoms, you will want to know the mode of delivery and the birth weight.

Sexual history

It is not usual to take a detailed sexual history in gynaecology but a limited sexual history may be appropriate and this information will determine if a more detailed history is required.

Social history

The usual details on smoking, alcohol and use of recreational/non-prescription drugs are useful. It is also important to know about social support and care for patients returning home after gynaecological surgery, particularly if the woman is responsible for the care of young children or elderly relatives.

Many gynaecological conditions are not life-threatening and therefore the impact of any condition on quality of life needs to be assessed. For example, a woman may be found to have asymptomatic fibroids or some degree of vaginal prolapse on attending for a smear test but if these are not reducing her quality of life, it is perfectly reasonable not to take further action.

Examination of the gynaecological patient

Women with a gynaecological complaint require a full examination but the aspects that are different to routine examination are abdominal and pelvic examination.

Abdominal examination

It is important to offer the patient privacy to undress and to expose only the relevant area. The abdomen needs to be exposed from the xiphisternum down to the symphysis pubis. It is normal to keep the pubic area covered. Abdominal examination comprises of inspection, palpation, percussion and auscultation.

Inspection

It is normal to look for presence of any obvious distension by a mass, striae and movement with respiration. It is important to look for scars from previous surgery. If the patient has a previous low transverse incision, you need to ensure that the covering sheet is lowered sufficiently to check below the patient's pubic hair line. Remember to check for any scars inside the umbilicus from laparoscopy.

Palpation

Before performing superficial and deep palpation, check with the patient if she has any areas of tenderness. Begin your palpation in the quadrant away from this and examine the tender area last. Remember that women of reproductive age may be referred to gynaecology with non-gynaecological conditions and you need to examine the whole of the patient's abdomen including upper abdomen and renal angles.

If you detect tenderness, check for signs of peritonism; rebound tenderness and guarding. If you identify abdominal distension, you need to consider ascites and check for shifting dullness and a fluid thrill.

Table C Abdominal and pelvic clinical findings.

Clinical finding	Example of abdominal finding	Example from pelvic finding
Contour		
Well defined	Full bladder	Pregnant uterus
Diffuse	Tumour infiltration of omentum	Endometriosis
Smooth and regular	Ovarian cyst or fibroid	Ovarian cyst or fibroid
Irregular and craggy	Ovarian cancer	Ovarian cancer
		Possibly endometriosis
Mobility		
Mobile	Ovarian cyst	Ovarian cyst or fibroid
Fixed	Ovarian cancer	Chronic PID, endometriosis or cancer
Percussion		
Dull	Fibroid uterus	
Hyper-resonant	Full bladder or ovarian cyst	
Shifting dullness	Ascites	

PID, pelvic inflammatory disease.

If you detect a mass, you should try to determine if it is abdominal or pelvic in origin. Pelvic masses rise above the pubic symphysis and the lower border cannot be palpated. You should be able to describe the mass both on abdominal and pelvic examination in the terms described in Table C.

Auscultation
Auscultation for bowel sounds is a normal part of abdominal examination.

Pelvic examination
Preparing the patient for a pelvic examination
It is essential to have a professional approach to pelvic examination to reassure the patient and to prevent unnecessary embarrassment. Before starting the examination ensure that the patient understands the purpose of the examination and the procedures that you are going to follow. It is usual to position the patient lying down supine with her head slightly raised. If she is on a bed or couch you should ask her to bring her feet up close to her bottom and let her knees fall out in order for you to gain adequate access to perform a speculum examination. Many clinics and wards provide a gynaecological examination couch where the patient's legs are supported in leg rests. The use of foot pedals allow you to lower or raise the bed and tilt the patient backwards to aid examination and access for any outpatient procedures or investigations. You need to consider any necessary adaptations to ensure your patent's comfort, e.g. if she has restricted mobility.

Inspection
It is important to examine the vulval area with an adequate light source. This will allow you to see if there are any local lesions such as atrophic changes in the postmenopausal woman, ulceration or obvious prolapse.

Speculum examination
The purpose of speculum examination is to examine the lower genital tract. The vagina has an anterior and a posterior vaginal wall which are normally in close contact. Inserting the speculum allows the vaginal walls to be pushed apart gently so the vaginal wall and the cervix can be inspected and any relevant procedures, such as taking a vaginal swab or cervical smear test, can be carried out. It is important to be familiar with the Cusco speculum (bivalve speculum; Fig. J).

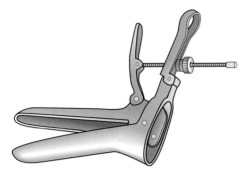

Figure J Cusco speculum.

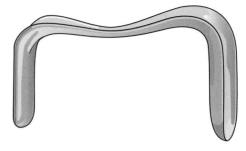

Figure K Sims speculum.

Practicalities of examining the patient
• Remember the General Medical Council (GMC) guidelines (Box A)
• Wash your hands either with soap and water or with alcohol rub
• Ensure your hands are completely dry before putting on your gloves; this helps you to put on your gloves smoothly
• Let the patient know when you are about to begin the examination and exactly what you are doing throughout the examination
• If using a metal speculum, ensure it is warm
• Assemble the speculum prior to the examination (unless you are using a pre-assembled disposable speculum)
• Apply only a small amount of lubricant jelly to the end of the speculum (large amounts will be wiped off on insertion leaving your patient messy)
• If you are obtaining a liquid-based cytology sample for cervical screening, the lubricant can cause cytolysis and you can just dip the speculum in normal saline

Speculum technique
• If you are right-handed you should hold the speculum in your right hand, keeping the anterior and posterior valves of the speculum closed.
• Use your left hand to separate the labia so the posterior fourchette is exposed. The most comfortable way to proceed is to insert the speculum directly, angling the speculum slightly down and back until fully inserted.
• The speculum should be inserted and opened slowly to avoid discomfort to your patient.
• If only inspection of the cervix and/or vagina is required then you can hold the blades of the speculum apart.

• If you need to perform any procedures, close the ratchet on a disposable plastic speculum or rotate the nut to the top to keep the speculum open.
• Asking your patient to cough can help to relax the pelvic floor and bring the cervix into view.

> **KEY POINT**
>
> Helping the patient to relax will aid your examination. It is useful to remind the patient not to hold her breath and to breathe slowly. Encourage your patient to think about pushing the speculum out as she exhales. This relaxes the pelvic floor and makes the examination less uncomfortable.

Removal of the speculum
Remember to withdraw the end of the speculum beyond the cervix before closing the blades together. Remove the speculum slowly and carefully.

When examining prolapse, a bivalve speculum holds both walls of the vagina apart. You need to use a Sims speculum (Fig. K) with the patient lying in the left lateral position.

Bimanual examination
The purpose of the bimanual examination is to examine the upper genital tract (uterus and adnexa). You should follow a systematic approach (Box B).

It is important to consider this examination in context as the signs that you are trying to elicit will be different in a patient presenting with acute pain from the patient seen in the gynaecology clinic. It is normal to perform a two finger examination using the index and middle finger with some lubricating jelly. In postmenopausal women, you should start with one finger to determine whether a two finger examination is possible or not.

Box B Objective structured clinical examination (OSCE) checklist for pelvic examination

Preliminarily introduce yourself	(1 mark)
Explain procedure to patient	(1 mark)
Explain rationale for performing a pelvic examination or explain to patient why pelvic examination needs to be carried out	(1 mark)
Obtain the patient's consent	(1 mark)
Offer chaperone or invite the patient to bring in a friend or relative	(1 mark)
Record consent and name of chaperone, give the patient privacy to dress and undress	(1 mark)
Avoid unnecessary personal comments	(1 mark)
Keep the discussion relevant	(1 mark)

Speculum technique

Wash hands before and after examination	(0-1-2 marks)
Assemble Cusco speculum correctly prior to examination	(1 mark)
Use small amount of lubricant	(1 mark)
Insert speculum correctly	(1 mark)
Open speculum and demonstrate cervix fully seen	(1 mark)
Explain procedure during examination	(1 mark)
Take care when removing the speculum and ensure patient's comfort	(1 mark)
Recover patient on completing examination	(1 mark)

Pelvic examination

Pelvic examination should not be performed in prepubescent girls or if there is a clinical contraindication. You should consider either a transabdominal ultrasound scan of the pelvis or examination under anaesthetic if necessary.

Vaginal examination

First feel the cervix:

• In a nulliparous patient, this is smooth, firm and regular

• In the parous patient, the normal cervix may be bulky, smoothly irregular with ectopy or formation of Nabothian follicles (blocked mucous glands)

Remember there is a wide normal range related to physiological changes including oestrogen levels and childbirth.

Bimanual palpation

The aim of bimanual examination is to palpate the uterus and possibly the adnexa between your examining hand

on the lower abdomen and your fingers in the vagina. Push up on the uterus vaginally with your fingers anterior to the cervix. Push down with the left hand over the lower abdominal wall. You should feel the uterus between both hands and note its size. It is usual to compare the size of the uterus in terms of weeks' gestation even in the non-pregnant patient. If you are unsure of this, try to visualize it in terms of the size of fruit:

• A small tangerine = 8 weeks
• A small orange = 10 weeks
• A large orange = 12 weeks
• A grapefruit = 14 weeks (and will be palpable just about the pubic symphysis on abdominal palpation)

If the uterus is enlarged, consider if it is generally enlarged (such as the bulky uterus of a parous patient or pregnancy) or if there is an obvious mass involving the uterus (such as fibroids).

Note if the uterus is anteverted or retroverted. If you cannot palpate the uterus, it may be retroverted. Note whether the uterus is mobile or fixed (Table C).

Examining the adnexae

Move the tips of your fingers into each lateral vaginal fornix at the side of the cervix in turn. Also palpate from above with your abdominal hand on the same side. Normal ovaries are only likely to be felt in a thin premenopausal woman. Palpation of an adnexal mass usually indicates that pathology is present. Ascertain whether any mass is smooth and regular or irregular and whether it is fixed or mobile (Table C). Use the bimanual technique to feel if a mass is attached to the uterus or separate. Remember that fixed irregular masses in the adnexa are more likely to be related to endometriosis or the effects of scarring from chronic pelvic inflammatory disease than malignancy. It is equally important to note if there is any tenderness on palpation of the adnexa. Check for cervical excitation (Box C).

Following examination

First allow the patient to dress herself. The changing area should give her privacy. Tissues to wipe away excess jelly and facilities for her to wash her hands should be provided. Clear away your examining instruments and wash your hands again. Once you have completed this, you should discuss your findings with the patient and your proposed plan for further investigations and management.

The obstetric patient

Most pregnant women are fit and healthy and will remain 'low risk' through the pregnancy and birth, with the midwife being the lead caregiver. However, there are some maternal conditions that predate pregnancy and some conditions arising during the pregnancy that can worsen maternal and/or fetal outcomes and need additional medical care. The main aim of antenatal care is to assess 'risk' to the mother and baby at every stage of the pregnancy and to offer appropriate investigations, with the overall aim of achieving a healthy baby and mother at the end of the pregnancy, and to make the pregnancy and birth a satisfying, fulfilling and happy journey for the parents.

Box C Cervical excitation

The equivalent in pelvic examination of rebound tenderness is to elicit cervical excitation (Fig. M). By pushing the cervix laterally this will stretch the adnexa on the same side of the pelvis as the uterus tilts to the opposite side (excitation elicited results from peritonism in the adnexa)

Causes of cervical excitation
- Bleeding from an ectopic pregnancy or from a haemorrhagic cyst
- Cyst fluid from a ruptured ovarian cyst
- Inflammation from a torted ovarian cyst or a tubovarian abscess

---

Preconception care

While most women will present when they are pregnant, care should ideally begin preconception, when a pregnancy is being planned. Folic acid is advised (to reduce the risk of fetal neural tube defects), as is advice regarding a healthier lifestyle including reducing or stopping smoking (see Case 20) and a healthy diet.

For some women, preconception care is especially important: for example, women with insulin-dependent diabetes (see Case 21), epilepsy, hypertension on angiotensin converting enzyme (ACE) inhibitors (see Case 21) or those with a previous history of pregnancy affected by open neural tube defect. In women with epilepsy not on medication, there is an increased risk of fetal abnormalities (4% vs a 3% risk in the general population), but this risk is further increased when the mother is on antiepileptic medications such as phenytoin or sodium valproate. These fetal abnormalities include cleft lip and palate, cardiac and neural tube defects. While the risk with one drug is around 6–7%, this risk increases with the number of antiepileptic drugs taken. The aim of prepregnancy care therefore is to achieve good seizure control on a single drug, if possible.

Similarly, in women who have been seizure-free for some years there may be the option of discontinuing antiepileptic medication. However, this must be

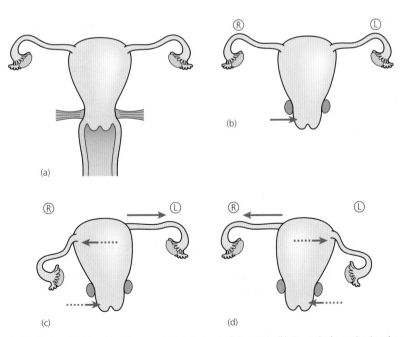

Figure L Eliciting cervical excitation. (a) The uterus is supported at the level of the cervix. (b) On vaginal examination the cervix is pushed to one side. (c) This pushes the uterus in the opposite direction, but puts the adnexa on stretch eliciting discomfort if excitiation is present. (d) The cervix should then be moved in the opposite direction.

considered and implemented only under appropriate physician or neurological advice and supervision. A higher dose of preconception folic acid supplementation of 5 mg is also advised (as in mothers with a previous pregnancy affected by neural tube defect).

In couples with known genetic problems (e.g. carriers of cystic fibrosis or sickle cell trait), counselling regarding the fetal risks of acquiring the disease and the invasive diagnostic tests (e.g. chorion villus sampling and amniocentesis) that might be available should ideally be discussed preconception.

Care in pregnancy
Dating of the pregnancy
Although pregnancy begins at conception, it is more convenient to date from the first day of a woman's last menstrual period (LMP). Naegele's rule estimates the expected date of delivery (EDD) from the first day of the woman's LMP by adding a year, subtracting 3 months and adding 7 days to that date. This approximates to the average human pregnancy which lasts 40 weeks (280 days) from the LMP, or 38 weeks (266 days) from the date of fertilization. Counting from the LMP, a term pregnancy usually lasts between 37 and 42 weeks.

As women may not accurately remember their LMP, or their menstrual cycles may not be very regular, dating of the pregnancy by the measurement of the crown–rump length as determined by a scan in the first trimester is thought to be more accurate. Determining the gestational age accurately is important, both in case the woman labours prematurely and if she goes postdated to help with induction of labour at the appropriate time.

Some obstetric definitions
Gravidity is defined as the number of times that a woman has been pregnant and *parity* is the number of pregnancies she has had with a gestational age of 24 weeks or more, regardless of whether the child was born alive or stillborn. There is usually a second number added on to parity which is the number of pregnancy losses before 24 weeks' gestation. Therefore, para 0 + 0 is a woman who has never been pregnant before. Para 1 + 1 implies one previous pregnancy beyond 24 weeks (live or stillbirth) + one pregnancy loss before 24 weeks (a termination, miscarriage or ectopic pregnancy). A women who is currently in her first pregnancy is gravida 1 para 0 (G1 P0) and a parous women with three previous term live births and two 10-week spontaneous miscarriages and

currently pregnant would be gravida 6 para 3 + 2 (G6 P3 + 2).

- *Term* gestation is usually 37–42 completed weeks' gestation
- *Preterm* is less than 37 weeks' gestation
- *Mildly preterm* is 32–36 weeks' gestation
- *Very preterm* is less than 32 weeks' gestation
- *Extremely preterm* is less than 28 weeks' gestation

Antenatal appointments
The needs of each pregnant woman should be assessed at the first booking appointment (which ideally should be in the first trimester) and reassessed at each appointment throughout pregnancy because new problems can arise at any time. A schedule of antenatal appointments should be determined by the degree of risk identified. In a nulliparous woman with an uncomplicated pregnancy, 10 appointments, and in a parous woman with an uncomplicated pregnancy, a schedule of seven antenatal visits is usually adequate. Generally, in a parous woman having gone through at least one previous uncomplicated pregnancy, it is easier to assign risk than in a nulliparous woman in her first pregnancy (Box D).

As with any other patient, assessment begins with taking an appropriate history at the booking visit. The general principles of approach to the patient are as described above in the gynaecology section.

History
History includes details of the mother and the current pregnancy to date including maternal age – young teenage mothers are at increased risk from preterm labour, and have an increased incidence of pre-eclampsia and small for gestational age babies. Scans to monitor fetal growth, more frequent blood pressure checks and education as to the signs and symptoms of preterm labour may be indicated.

With increasing maternal age the risk of chromosomal abnormalities such as trisomy 21 increases and also the incidence of hypertension and type 2 diabetes. Invasive prenatal genetic tests available for confirming fetal karyotype (see Case 20) may need to be discussed; regular monitoring of blood pressure and consideration of an oral glucose tolerance test are also indicated.

Present pregnancy
What is her estimated gestation from the last menstrual period (gestational age and viability is best confirmed by a first trimester scan) and has she has been well thus far

Box D An example of schedule of routine antenatal care

First contact with a health care professional
(ideally should be preconception)
Evaluate history/risk factors

Discussion should include:
- Folic acid supplementation
- Food hygiene, including how to reduce the risk of a food-acquired infection
- Lifestyle advice, including smoking cessation, recreational drug use and alcohol consumption
- All antenatal screening, including risks and benefits of the screening tests

Booking appointment *(ideally by 10 weeks)*
- Evaluate 'risk' (including evaluation of social and domestic circumstances) and women who need additional care and plan pattern of care for the pregnancy
- Offer early ultrasound scan for gestational age assessment
- Check blood group and rhesus D status
- Offer screening for haemoglobinopathies (if indicated), anaemia, red cell alloantibodies, hepatitis B virus, HIV, rubella susceptibility and syphilis infection
- Offer screening for asymptomatic bacteriuria
- Inform pregnant women younger than 25 years about the high prevalence of *Chlamydia* infection in their age group and offer screening
- Offer screening for Down's syndrome
- Offer mid-trimester ultrasound screening for structural anomalies
- Measure height, weight and calculate body mass index
- Measure blood pressure and test urine for proteinuria
- Offer screening for gestational diabetes (in the 'at risk' group)
- Evaluate mood to identify possible depression

16 weeks
- Discuss the results of all screening tests undertaken
- Investigate a haemoglobin level below 110 g/L and consider iron supplementation if indicated
- Measure blood pressure and test urine for proteinuria

18–20 weeks
Mid-trimester anomaly scan if the woman chooses to have this

24–25 weeks *(for nulliparous women)*
- Measure symphysiofundal height
- Measure blood pressure and test urine for proteinuria

28 weeks
- Offer a second screening for anaemia and atypical red cell alloantibodies

- If haemoglobin level below 105 g/L, consider iron supplementation, if indicated
- Offer anti-D prophylaxis to rhesus-negative women
- Blood pressure and urine for proteinuria
- Measure symphysiofundal height

31–32 weeks *(nulliparous women)*
- Blood pressure and urine for proteinuria
- Measure symphysiofundal height

34 weeks
- Discussion of antenatal classes in preparation for labour and birth, including pain relief in labour and the birth plan
- Offer a second dose of anti-D to rhesus-negative women
- Blood pressure and urine for proteinuria
- Measure symphysiofundal height

36 weeks
- Discuss vitamin K prophylaxis and newborn infant screening tests, postnatal care, awareness of baby blues and postnatal depression
- Blood pressure and urine for proteinuria
- Measure symphysiofundal height, check lie/position of baby
- If baby in the breech presentation, offer external cephalic version

38 weeks
- Blood pressure and urine for proteinuria
- Measure symphysiofundal height, check lie/position of baby
- Information of prolonged pregnancy including its management

40 weeks
- Blood pressure and urine for proteinuria
- Measure symphysiofundal height, check lie/position of baby

41 weeks
For women undelivered by 41 weeks:
- A membrane sweep should be offered
- Induction of labour should be offered
- Measure blood pressure and test urine for proteinuria
- Measure symphysiofundal height

At each visit, 'risk' (including that relating to domestic abuse, mood changes) must be assessed and care planned accordingly

(any history of bleeding, nausea, vomiting or urinary symptoms)? Is there any particular presenting complaint? Is she on folic acid?

Previous obstetric history

A careful history for each of the woman's previous pregnancies should be sought. This includes details of the antenatal course, gestation at and mode of delivery, birth weight of the baby and his/her condition at birth.

Antenatal complications

Details of antenatal complications including pre-eclampsia, antepartum haemorrhage, preterm prelabour rupture of membranes, venous thrombosis, cholestasis of pregnancy, intrauterine fetal growth restriction (IUGR), stillbirth and congenital abnormality are important. In a woman with the same partner who has had pre-eclampsia in her first pregnancy there is an approximate 8–10% risk of recurrence. In women with early onset severe pre-eclampsia or those with severe fetal growth restriction, especially if recurrent, the option of low dose aspirin could be discussed. With a previous history of cholestasis of pregnancy, the recurrence risk might range around 40–80% (with a 30–40% risk of having pruritus while on the oral combined contraceptive pill) and plans to monitor the clinical symptoms, liver function tests including bile acid estimations and fetal well-being can be put in place.

Labour and delivery

Details regarding the labour and delivery including whether the labour was induced or spontaneous, gestation at delivery; a previous preterm labour puts a mother at a higher risk of this again. If the labour was quick and painless (or it was a second trimester painless pregnancy loss), the differential diagnosis of an 'incompetent' cervix should be borne in mind. Cervical assessment with ultrasound in the second trimester may be indicated, with the option of insertion of a cervical suture if the cervix shows signs of funnelling or shortening. Similarly, with a history of recurrent preterm labours there might be a place for prophylactic administration of steroids for fetal lung maturity at a reasonable gestation before the anticipated start of labour (although this is not easy to predict).

Mode of delivery

See Case 23.

Details of the third stage

Details of the third stage including any history of postpartum haemorrhage (PPH), third degree tears, manual removal of the placenta under an anaesthetic should be sought. Some of these have a higher risk of recurrence (especially if they have occurred on two or more occasions) and prophylactic third stage management with oxytocin or syntometrine may be indicated.

Details of the neonate

Details of the neonate including birth weight and condition at birth, especially if requiring admission to the neonatal unit, should be sought.

Puerperium

A history of any problems in the puerperium should be sought including sepsis, secondary PPH and depression. Especially with postpartum depression/psychosis, plans should be in place for careful assessment of the woman's mood both antenatally and postnatally, with access to adequate support and help.

Medical and surgical history

This is an important aspect of an antenatal history as there may be conditions that affect the pregnancy or that the pregnancy could change with either deterioration (e.g. cardiac disease) or improvement (e.g. some autoimmune disorders) or an alteration in treatment or dosage might be indicated (e.g. with ACE antihypertensives, or with thyroxine replacement in hypothyroidism where often an increase in dose through the pregnancy is required). Multidisciplinary team care, involving the cardiologist, haematologist, rheumatologist and endocrinologist as the case demands, may need to be planned for. A complete drug history (including over-the-counter prescriptions) is also essential (e.g. high dose vitamin A may be teratogenic in the first trimester).

Gynaecological history

• This should include the menstrual history – the regularity and pattern of previous menstrual cycles, the LMP
• Previous contraceptive use
• Cervical smear history – if a smear is due this can be performed in early pregnancy, but it might be preferable to wait till past the puerperium if there has no previous concerning smear history
• Any other relevant history (e.g. of pelvic inflammatory disease, sexually transmitted disease)

Family history

A history of consanguinity, of genetic or familial syndromes, is important to be able to organize appropriate counselling and tests if available. Some conditions such as diabetes, pre-eclampsia and cholestasis are seen more often in women who have a familial history of these.

Social history

A history of smoking, alcohol use and any other substance misuse should be probed as these could affect pregnancy. Excessive alcohol use could cause fetal effects spanning the spectrum of fetal alcohol syndrome from mild to severe (e.g. microcephaly, midface hypoplasia, flat philtrum, cardiac abnormalities, learning and developmental delay). Opiate and cocaine substance misuse increase the risk of preterm labour, IUGR, antepartum haemorrhage, fetal distress and neonatal abstinence syndrome, with cocaine especially increasing the risk of placental abruption. With intravenous drug use there is also the higher incidence of maternal infections such as hepatitis B and C and of venous thrombosis.

This group of vulnerable women require targeted multidisciplinary antenatal care involving the substance misuse services to stabilize drug use (mostly with prescribed oral methadone), prevent substance withdrawal (which increases the risk of preterm labour and fetal distress), screening for infections and surveillance of the baby.

It is also an important part of antenatal assessment to evaluate if the baby will be going into a safe and appropriate environment and if additional help is needed to achieve this.

Antenatal appointments should include measuring body mass index (BMI) at the booking appointment and blood pressure (BP) and testing urine for proteinuria and ketones. The offer of the following screening tests should be made:
• Early ultrasound scan for confirming viability, gestational age and whether a singleton or multiple pregnancy
• Blood group and rhesus D (RhD) status
• Screening for anaemia, red cell alloantibodies, hepatitis B virus, HIV, rubella susceptibility and syphilis infection
• Screening for asymptomatic bacteriuria
• Screening for Down's syndrome
• Ultrasound screening for structural anomalies (20 s)

For certain women additional tests may be offered; for example, *Chlamydia* testing in the under 25s, a haemoglobinopathy screen in those of African or Mediterranean descent (to look for sickle cell or thalassaemia carriers). At around 28 weeks repeat red cell alloantibody screening and a haemoglobin recheck are offered. Screening for gestational diabetes varies from centre to centre and may include a random glucose check on all women

at some point in the early third trimester to an oral glucose tolerance test (OGTT) when risk factors are identified in the history (e.g. previous large for dates baby, family history of diabetes, Asian origin, increased BMI) or examination (e.g. polyhydramnios, large baby or recurrent glycosuria in current pregnancy; see Case 21).

Women should be informed about the purpose of any screening test before it is performed, and should have the option to accept or decline a test (Box E).

Box E Conditions increasing maternal and/or fetal risks

Examples of conditions in pregnant women increasing their pregnancy risks, with obstetric and/or medical care indicated:
• Cardiac disease
• Hypertension
• Renal disease
• Endocrine disorder or diabetes requiring insulin
• Psychiatric disorder (on medication)
• Haematological disorder, including thromboembolic disease
• Autoimmune diseases such as antiphospholipid syndrome
• Epilepsy requiring anticonvulsant drugs
• Severe asthma
• Drug use such as heroin, cocaine (including crack cocaine) and ecstasy
• HIV or hepatitis B virus infection
• Obesity (BMI of 35 or more at first contact) or underweight (BMI less than 18 at first contact)

Women who have experienced any of the following in previous pregnancies
• Recurrent miscarriage (three or more consecutive pregnancy losses) or a mid-trimester loss
• Severe pre-eclampsia, HELLP syndrome or eclampsia
• Rhesus isoimmunization or other significant blood group antibodies
• Uterine surgery including caesarean section, myomectomy
• Antenatal or postpartum haemorrhage on two occasions
• Retained placenta on two occasions
• Puerperal psychosis
• Grand multiparity (more than six pregnancies)
• A stillbirth or neonatal death
• A small for gestational age infant (<5th centile)
• A large for gestational age infant (>95th centile)
• A baby weighing <2500 g or >4500 g
• A baby with a congenital anomaly (structural or chromosomal)

Examination

General examination

It is good practice to start with a general examination, remembering the normal physiological changes that do occur from very early on in the pregnancy. Checking for pallor, peripheral odema, jaundice and dehydration if there is increased vomiting, and where indicated for varicose veins, thyroid enlargement and tendon reflexes are important.

Blood pressure in pregnancy should be measured appropriately. The woman should be relaxed, semi-recumbent at about a 30° angle and the blood pressure should be measured with an appropriately sized cuff (the width of the cuff should be 40% of the arm circumference) from her right arm at the level of the heart. Women with a high BMI may need a larger cuff. While systolic blood pressure is when the Korotkoff's sounds are first heard, there has been much controversy as to whether the muffling or disappearance of sounds should be taken for diastolic blood pressure. The general consensus from obstetricians based on careful analysis of the evidence is that disappearance of sounds (fifth phase) is the most accurate measurement of diastolic pressure, with the proviso that in those rare instances in which sounds persist to zero the fourth phase of muffling of sounds should be used.

Abdominal examination

As with any other examination, a structured approach is best.

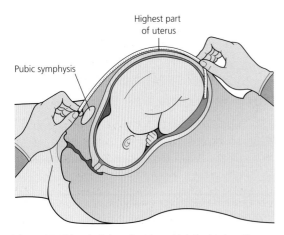

Highest part
of uterus

Pubic symphysis

Figure M Mid-sagittal view of mother with baby *in utero*. The fundal height is determined by measuring the distance from the pubic symphysis to the highest part of the uterus. A 33-week baby should measure 33 cm (+/– 3 cm).

Inspection includes determining the degree of distension of the abdomen and to see if it generally appears appropriate to the period of gestation (e.g. does it appear overdistended with umbilical eversion – this might be seen with multiple pregnancy, polyhydramnios or fetal marcosomia), for any fetal movements that may be obvious, the presence of old or new striae gravidarum and linea nigra, and for any scars of previous surgery (of previous caesarean section, laparotomy, laparoscopy or appendicectomy).

Before palpating, it is good practice to enquire if the woman has been in any pain. The fundus of the uterus is palpated with the ulnar border of the hand by gradually palpating down from the xiphisternum until the fundus is reached. The symphysiofundal height (SFH) is then measured from the upper border of the symphysis pubis to the fundus, in centimetres (Fig. M).

This is routine screening for fetal growth problems; generally, +/– 3 cm from the period of gestation, especially in the third trimester, may indicate a large for dates or a small for date fetus, respectively. This needs to be confirmed by a fetal growth scan in most cases as SFH is not a very sensitive or specific examination tool.

Fundal palpation may help to determine if the fetal breech or head is at the fundus. Lateral palpation helps determine the lie (longitudinal, oblique or transverse) of the fetus and where the back and limbs might be. Both hands are placed flat on either side of the abdomen and the fetus is gently balloted between the two to feel the fetal back and limbs. An attempt must be made to assess the liquor volume – in oligohydramnios fetal parts may be very clearly felt while with polyhydramnios the opposite is the case (Fig. N).

The presenting part is then palpated with both hands on either side of the lower pole of the uterus to confirm if it is the head or the breech presenting and then to determine if it is engaged (widest presenting part through the pelvic inlet). This is also commented on as how many fifths of the head can be felt per abdomen – generally when a head is engaged with it is palpable two-fifths or less per abdomen.

The fetal heart is then heard through a Doppler Sonicaid or, increasingly less so these days, with a Pinard stethoscope. The site for the most appropriate check of the fetal heart is easier if the lie of the fetus, its back and presenting part are clearly identified with the abdominal palpation.

Uterine tenderness on palpation may be elicited in cases of chorioamnionitis (see Case 19), placental

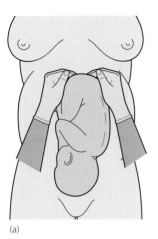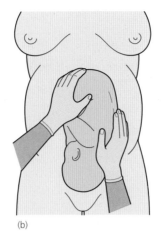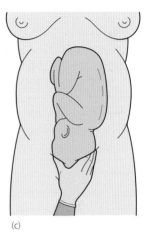

(a)   (b)   (c)

Figure N Abdominal palpation. (a) Fundal palpation to ascertain the fetal part at the fundus. (b) Lateral palpation to determine the lie (longitudinal, oblique or transverse). (c) Palpation to determine whether presenting part engaged in maternal pelvis.

abruption (see Case 18) and degeneration of uterine fibroids. There may be epigastric pain and tenderness over the liver in HELLP (haemolytic anaemia, elevated liver enzymes and low platelet count; see Case 16). There may be other non-obstetric causes of painful abdomen including reflux, urinary tract infection, appendicitis, torsion of an ovarian cyst and gall stones, and appropriate history, examination and investigations should be evaluated to make a diagnosis. The pregnant uterus could alter some classic clinical signs; for example, tenderness over the McBurney point or rebound tenderness in appendicitis may not be elicited because of displacement of the appendix from its normal position.

When examining for uterine contractions in labour, the strength of the contraction (mild, moderate, strong), the frequency (how many contractions in 10 minutes) and if the uterus is relaxing well between contractions must all be taken into account. A uterus that is contracting more than five times in 10 minutes without adequate relaxation between contractions (with each contraction lasting more than 1 minute) can be described as having tachysystole, and if this is associated with fetal heart rate abnormalities it is labelled as hyperstimulation (hyperstimulation also includes a sustained uterine contraction ≥2 minutes). These features are especially important when monitoring for side-effects of prostaglandin induction of labour and oxytocin augmentation of labour.

Vaginal examination

Vaginal examinations are not very often indicated antenatally, although they are very important in labour to assess progress. Some of the indications for an antenatal vaginal speculum examination are as follow:
• To confirm preterm premature rupture of membranes (PPROM; see Case 19)
• To look for local causes of antepartum bleeding after a scan has ruled out a low-lying placenta (see Case 17)
• To perform swabs when there is a history of symptomatic vaginal discharge
• Where there may be a threatened miscarriage or preterm labour
• Occasionally, to perform a cervical smear
A digital examination may be indicated to:
• Confirm cervical changes of labour – both in preterm and term labour
• Evaluate the ripeness of the cervix (Bishop's score; see Case 14) to determine if prostaglandin ripening is indicated when induction of labour is planned
• For sweeping of membranes in postdated pregnancies prior to formal induction of labour
• Evaluate progress in labour (see Case 14)

All the principles of performing an intimate examination and the techniques are as described above in the section on the gynaecological patient. Generally, in pregnancy the cervix looks somewhat different from that in the non-pregnant state; it is softer, appears larger and more vascular, and may have a large ectropion (usually a normal physiological change of pregnancy). The internal os may be more difficult to visualize especially as the pregnancy progresses as a result of the growing uterus altering its normal position, and there may be a greater amount of the normal physiological vaginal discharge.

In conclusion, good antenatal care involves risk assessment; this has to be ongoing through the pregnancy as the level of risk could change at any stage (and during labour, delivery and puerperium). Risk assessment is based on a combination of past obstetric and maternal medical, surgical, family, social and drug history, maternal demographics such as age and BMI, the results of routine examination (e.g. increase in BP suggesting pregnancy induced hypertension or pre-eclamptic toxaemia, or a lower SFH suggesting IUGR) and the results of antenatal screening tests.

References

Antenatal care: routine care for the healthy pregnant woman. NICE Clinical Guideline CG62. March 2008.

GMC Guidelines on Intimate Examination: Maintaining Boundaries. November 2006.

A 24-year-old woman with vaginal bleeding in early pregnancy

Anna Smith, a 24-year-old para 0+1 is brought in to the early pregnancy assessment unit by her husband with fresh vaginal bleeding. Her last period was 6 weeks ago. She is very anxious as she had a similar episode in a previous pregnancy and miscarried.

What should you do on initial assessment?

You need to ensure that Mrs Smith is haemodynamically stable. This initial assessment follows the basic principles of ABC. You must assess her bleeding. If she is bleeding heavily and is tachycardic or hypotensive then IV access should be obtained along with fluid replacement before obtaining a detailed history.

What differential diagnosis immediately comes to mind?

- Miscarriage
- Delayed period
- Ectopic pregnancy
- Molar pregnancy
- Cervical lesion

What would you like to elicit from the history?
History of presenting complaint

1 Bleeding
   a. Amount and colour of bleeding
   b. History of passage of any fleshy tissues/clots
   c. How long she has been bleeding?
2 Pain
   a. Is bleeding associated with pain?
   b. Site, severity, type and radiation of pain
   c. History of shoulder tip pain

3 About menstrual cycle
   a. When was her last menstrual period?
   b. How regular were the cycles?
   c. Was she planning the pregnancy?
   d. Has she carried out a pregnancy test?
4 Contraceptive history
5 Previous obstetric history
Outcome of the previous pregnancy (miscarriage, ectopic)
6 Past history
   a. Previous pelvic inflammatory disease
   b. Sexually transmitted infections

Mrs Smith tells you that she had noticed fresh red blood which was only spotting on wiping herself. It was associated with cramping lower abdominal pain. She describes the pain as mild in intensity, non-radiating and present for the last hour. She has not taken any analgesic as yet. A urine pregnancy test which she did at home 2 days ago was positive. She has a regular κ = 5/30–35 day cycle. Her last period was 6 weeks ago.

Her previous pregnancy was a spontaneous conception 8 months ago. Unfortunately, she had a miscarriage at 7 weeks after an episode of spotting at 6 weeks' gestation. She is terrified that this is going to happen again. She and her partner have been trying to conceive since her last miscarriage.

What would you look for in physical examination?
General examination

Pallor, tachycardia and hypotension can be found with very heavy bleeding but this is uncommon.

Abdominal examination

After your initial assessment, you need to do an abdominal examination to detect any palpable mass. Any point of tenderness, guarding or rigidity should be elicited. Tenderness and guarding can be present in cases of

Obstetrics and Gynaecology: Clinical Cases Uncovered.
By M. Cruickshank and A. Shetty. Published 2009 by Blackwell Publishing. ISBN 978-1-4051-8671-1.

ectopic pregnancy because of intraperitoneal bleeding. Molar pregnancy can present with uterine size more than the period of gestation but is now usually diagnosed on ultrasound scan before this stage.

Pelvic examination

Look for signs of bleeding and assess how much she is bleeding. If she is wearing a pad, note if the pad is soaked or if her underwear is stained. You should note if there is active bleeding with blood trickling as this is a sign of a significant bleed.

Speculum examination

- Gently insert the speculum and see if there is bleeding in the vagina
- Use a sponge on sponge holder to see if there is any fresh bleeding
- If bleeding is seen you need to identify if it is heavy
- Check the cervical os:
  ○ look to see whether the external os is open or closed
  ○ look for any products of conception
- Check for any local lesion such as a polyp or cervical erosion

What is the clinical significance of the cervical os and the bleeding?
Inevitable miscarriage

There is persistent bleeding. Ballooning of the cervix results from products of conception in the cervical canal and the external os is open. The process is inevitable miscarriage and this is irreversible.

Incomplete miscarriage

There is a history of heavier bleeding with passage of clots or products of conception. The external os is open and products can be removed.

Missed miscarriage (early fetal demise)

If bleeding is present, it is likely to be a dark brown discharge and the os is closed. This may also be the situation in ectopic pregnancy.

Now review your clinical findings.

She had her last miscarriage when she was on holiday, and no hospital records are available. At present she is haemodynamically stable. She does not look pale and her pulse is 70 beats/minute. She is up to date with her cervical smears and the last one, taken 2 months ago, was reported as normal.

Her uterus is not palpable on abdominal examination. There is tenderness in the suprapubic area but there is no guarding or rigidity. The cervical os is closed and there is a small amount of fresh blood on her pad. No further bleeding can be seen from the external os. Her cervix is long with no evidence of ballooning. Bimanual examination does not reveal any mass or tenderness.

What investigations would you do?

1 *Full blood count.* A full blood count will assess if she has had a significant blood loss.
2 *Blood group and save.* Because she had her last miscarriage elsewhere we do not have any records of her blood group. You need to identify if she is rhesus negative as if she has further heavy bleeding she may require transfusion.

To summarize findings so far, Mrs Smith is spontaneously pregnant for the second time with 6 weeks' amenorrhoea, vaginal bleeding and lower abdomen pain. There is no history of passage of clots or products of conception. Her pregnancy test is positive. She is haemodynamically stable. Pelvic examination reveals no active bleeding and a closed cervical os. There is no abdominal tenderness, guarding or rigidity.

What will you do next?

An ultrasound scan of her pelvis. This should be transvaginal to obtain a clear view of the uterine cavity and its contents at her early gestation. You should warn her that we might not be able to see a pregnancy even with a transvaginal scan, even if it is intrauterine, because of her early gestation. Although she gives a history of 6 weeks' amenorrhoea, she may be only 5 weeks' pregnant as her cycle length is 30–35 days. Explain that transvaginal ultrasound is not harmful to pregnancy and by itself will not cause a miscarriage.

Pelvic ultrasound scan

A viable pregnancy can be seen from 5 weeks by transvaginal scan. A pelvic ultrasound scan of the pelvis is helpful in ruling out ectopic pregnancy. The presence of an intrauterine pregnancy almost always rules out ectopic pregnancy. There is a 1 in 40,000 chance of a heterotrophic pregnancy (both an intrauterine and an extrauterine pregnancy) in a spontaneous conception.

Box 1.1 Early embryology

Implantation in the uterine cavity occurs around cycle day 21, once the blastocyst enters the uterine cavity. Once the blastocyst comes in contact with decidualized endometrium, the trophoblast proliferates and differentiates into two layers: cytotrophoblast and syncytiotrophoblast (cells in contact with endometrium). Two layers of cytotrophoblast are separated by extraembryonic mesoderm

Gestational sac

A gestational sac is usually imaged as a round or oval anechoeic structure and can be seen as early as 20–23 days after ovulation. This develops from isolated spaces in the extraembryonic mesoderm fusing and forming a simple fluid-filled cavity that contains amnion, yolk sac and embryo

Yolk sac

Yolk sac, a spherical structure, develops on cycle day 28, when the extracoelomic membrane extends completely around the inner wall of the blastocyst forming a secondary cavity. It can be seen on transvaginal scan by 5 weeks. When present, the yolk sac confirms the diagnosis of intrauterine pregnancy

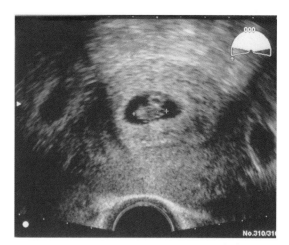

Figure 1.1 Pelvic ultrasound scan of an intrauterine pregnancy.

What ultrasound features would you look for to diagnose a pregnancy-related cause for her bleeding?

Ectopic pregnancy

If the uterine cavity is empty or if there is no definite sign of intrauterine pregnancy (presence of at least a yolk sac or fetal pole), you need to consider ectopic pregnancy. A pseudogestational intrauterine sac is seen in 10–20% of cases of ectopic pregnancy. There is a collection of fluid inside the uterine cavity as a result of inflammatory reaction to the pregnancy hormones. There are subtle differentiating signs like contour of the sac, presence of a double ring and eccentric position which favours the diagnosis of a true sac rather than a pseudosac. However, the presence of a yolk sac is a sign of true intrauterine gestational sac and therefore intrauterine pregnancy. Other features of ectopic pregnancy on ultrasound are a complex adnexal cystic mass and free fluid in the peritoneal cavity (Box 1.1).

Ultrasound features of a viable pregnancy

In addition to the presence of an intrauterine gestation sac with yolk sac and fetal pole, there should be presence of a fetal heart (seen pulsating) to call it a viable pregnancy.

Ultrasound features of molar pregnancy

The uterus is enlarged in size and reveals the classic snowstorm appearance of mixed echogenic appearance indicating hydropic villi and intrauterine haemorrhage. The β human chorionic gonadotrophin (βHCG) level can be markedly raised. Large benign theca lutein cysts (caused by ovarian stimulation with βHCG) are seen in 20% of cases.

KEY POINT

An empty uterus on scan might represent a complete miscarriage, very early intrauterine pregnancy or an ectopic pregnancy

Her pelvic ultrasound scan reveals a thickened endometrium. A very small 2-mm sac is seen which cannot be differentiated from a pseudosac. There was no evidence of fetal pole or yolk sac. Her right ovary is normal and the left ovary shows a 2 × 2.5 cm cyst. There is minimal free fluid in the pouch of Douglas and an ectopic pregnancy cannot be ruled out.

Can you explain her pelvic scan findings?

You cannot detect a definite sign of intrauterine pregnancy. It may be that it is a very early pregnancy or an

> **Box 1.2 β subunit of human chorionic gonadotrophin**
>
> - This is a glycoprotein consisting of α and β subunits secreted by trophoblast tissue which gives us an idea of where the pregnancy is
> - The βHCG should double in 48 hours in cases of an ongoing intrauterine pregnancy
> - It rises, but less than double, in ectopic pregnancy (66%)
> - If it falls to half in 48 hours it suggests miscarriage
> - In 15% of normal intrauterine pregnancy the βHCG will rise less than double
> - In 15% of ectopic pregnancies, a doubling will be seen in 48 hours
> - Failure of βHCG to double in absence of an intrauterine pregnancy suggests the diagnosis of ectopic pregnancy
> - In cases of molar pregnancy, very high levels of βHCG can be seen
> - When considering the test results, the whole clinical situation must be taken into consideration

ectopic pregnancy. The cyst in the left ovary is probably a corpus luteum. Hence you need to investigate further.

What further investigation would you do now?

Although she has a positive urinary pregnancy test, an ectopic pregnancy cannot be ruled out on ultrasound and a serum βHCG is advised.

Explain to her the rationale for a serum βHCG?

See Box 1.2.

Now review her test results

βHCG result shows a value of 412 IU/L and her blood group result shows that she is group O rhesus negative. Her full blood count is normal.

What information do you need to give to her?

- Despite high resolution ultrasound, you may not be able to see evidence of intrauterine pregnancy at transvaginal ultrasound scan as the levels of βHCG are less than 1000 IU/L
- A level of 1000 IU/L is taken as a discriminatory level to be able to see an intrauterine gestation sac

- A repeat βHCG in 48 hours will help in this case to determine whether it is an ongoing pregnancy or not
- A single βHCG gives very limited information unless the levels are high

What is the clinical significance of her being rhesus negative?

Non-sensitized rhesus-negative women need to receive anti-D immunoglobulin in the following situations to prevent the development of anti-rhesus antibodies:
- Ectopic pregnancy
- All miscarriages over 12 weeks' gestation (including threatened)
- All miscarriages where the uterus is evacuated (whether medically or surgically)
- Threatened miscarriage under 12 weeks' gestation only when bleeding is heavy or associated with pain
- Complete miscarriage under 12 weeks' gestation only when there is formal intervention to evacuate the uterus

Does Anna require anti-D immunoglobulin?

She does not need anti-D immunoglobulin in her present situation but once a diagnosis has been made this may need to be reviewed. She can go home and return after 48 hours.

She returns 48 hours later for a repeat βHCG having had a further episode of spotting in the morning. The repeat blood test shows a value of 880 IU/L.

Review all your differential diagnoses

Threatened miscarriage. This is the most likely diagnosis so far. There is only a small amount of bleeding, the cervical os is closed and βHCG has doubled in 48 hours.

Inevitable miscarriage. Incomplete miscarriage means that the process of miscarriage has started and some products of conception have been expelled while the rest still remains. This is unlikely in this case as the os is closed and bleeding has stopped (apart from one episode of spotting). In inevitable miscarriage, women continue to experience cramping abdominal pain as the uterus is contracting and trying to expel the products. Moreover, the bleeding continues, gradually becoming heavier and you would see an open os on speculum examination. Although threatened miscarriage can progress to inevitable miscarriage, at present in this case there are no such signs.

Incomplete miscarriage. This is unlikely as Mrs Smith does not give a history of passing clots or products of conception. Moreover, the βHCG has doubled, indicating it is an ongoing pregnancy. In the case of miscarriage it should decrease, ideally to half in 48 hours. There is a risk of infection if products are left.

Complete miscarriage. This could be a possibility as the cervical os is closed and bleeding has stopped. However, there is no history of passage of clots or products of conception.

Missed miscarriage. This was a possibility initially but it was ruled out with the doubling βHCG. As the pregnancy stops growing, the βHCG levels will reduce. The symptoms of pregnancy may disappear.

Recurrent miscarriage. This is defined as the loss of three or more pregnancies consecutively. It affects 1% of women. In this case there is only one previous miscarriage, hence investigations for recurrent miscarriage (karyotype of both partners; lupus anticoagulant; anticardiolipin antibodies; thrombophilia screen) are not needed.

Ectopic pregnancy. Although initially plausible, this is unlikely as βHCG is doubled in 48 hours and there are no risk factors for ectopic pregnancy (previous ectopic, history of pelvic inflammatory diseases). Moreover, Anna is haemodynamically stable and there is no abdominal guarding and rigidity. However, it cannot be excluded until an intrauterine pregnancy is demonstrated on ultrasound.

Molar pregnancy. βHCG is too low for it to be a molar pregnancy, her uterus is not enlarged inappropriately to the period of gestation and there is no history of passing vesicles.

Bleeding from a local lesion. This has been excluded as there is no evidence of cervical ectopy or polyp on examination.

What would you tell this patient?

• You should reassure her because her serum βHCG has doubled in 48 hours
• It is most likely an early ongoing intrauterine pregnancy as she may be only 5 weeks' pregnant considering her 30–35 day cycle
• Ultrasound scan is not useful at present as the values of βHCG are still less than 1000 IU/L
• She should be advised to come back in a week's time for an ultrasound scan
• A 24-hour contact number for the early pregnancy assessment unit should be given in case she has further questions
• Further support should be offered as the couple are very anxious
• You need to explain to her that one miscarriage is very common. Up to 15–20% of pregnancies miscarry
• Investigations for miscarriage are not advised until a couple has had at least three consecutive miscarriages
• One miscarriage does not alter the outcome in future pregnancies

Anna returns in a week and her pelvic ultrasound now shows a single intrauterine gestation sac with yolk sac and fetal pole with a heart beat present.

What is the outlook now?

Her scan has confirmed a continuing intrauterine pregnancy. She will need more reassurance at least until her scan after 8 weeks, which is beyond the gestation of her last miscarriage. She should have a 24-hour contact number in case she bleeds heavily. Approximately 15% of pregnancies are complicated by a threatened miscarriage.

PART 2: CASES

CASE REVIEW

This case of a very anxious couple is typical of women who present with very light bleeding in very early pregnancy. Her reason for anxiety is primarily because of her previous history of miscarriage. At every stage in history-taking and examination it is important to remember that she wishes something to be done to prevent miscarriage happening again.

Despite her history it is important to rule out other causes of early pregnancy bleeding. History, examination and investigations in this case revealed a likely diagnosis of threatened miscarriage, although ectopic pregnancy could

not be ruled out until the intrauterine pregnancy was demonstrated. Although transvaginal ultrasound can demonstrate intrauterine pregnancy from 5½ weeks onwards, sometimes dates are mistaken and hence the actual period of gestation when prior menstrual cycles have been longer (30–35 days in this case).

There is no reason to keep her in hospital and an outpatient management is justified. Admission will not prevent the miscarriage if it were to occur again. She has been given a 24-hour contact number in case of heavy bleeding or pain.

KEY POINTS

- ABC of resuscitation forms the initial assessment for bleeding in pregnancy
- Ectopic pregnancy needs to be excluded in women with pain or bleeding in early pregnancy
- Ectopic pregnancy and miscarriage can present without the patient even realizing that she is pregnant
- Understand that psychological support is equally important as the medical management of the condition

- Follow-up for counselling may be required, especially as this is a repeat episode
- Support groups, a point of contact and follow-up reassurance scans will be needed
- Investigations for recurrent miscarriages are not warranted unless there are three consecutive miscarriages
- Even after two miscarriages there is 80% chance of having a live baby

Case 2 A 25-year-old woman presenting as an emergency with low abdominal pain

Kenzi Anderson is a 25-year-old woman who presents to the gynaecology ward as an emergency admission. She complains of lower abdominal pain which started 2 days ago and has become progressively worse. Although she complains of feeling sore across the lower part of her abdomen, the pain is worse on the left side.

What is the first thought that comes to mind which would influence your differential diagnoses?

Is this patient pregnant?

If pregnant, what would be your differential diagnosis?

- Ectopic pregnancy
- Miscarriage – threatened/incomplete/septic
- Rupture of corpus luteal cyst
- Haemorrhage into corpus luteal cyst

And if she is not pregnant?

- Acute pelvic inflammatory disease (PID)
- Ovarian cysts (haemorrhage or rupture)
- Ovarian cyst torsion
- Endometriosis
- Uterine fibroid degeneration
- Primary dysmenorrhoea
- Mittelschmerz
- Pelvic vein congestion

Do not forget other (non-gynaecological) causes of acute pelvic pain

- Gastrointestinal
- Urological

Obstetrics and Gynaecology: Clinical Cases Uncovered.
By M. Cruickshank and A. Shetty. Published 2009 by Blackwell Publishing. ISBN 978-1-4051-8671-1.

- Trauma
- Sickle cell crisis
- Mesenteric vascular occlusion

What would you like to elicit from the history?

Period of amenorrhoea

Be wary that the patient may be pregnant.

History of presenting complaint

- Frequency, duration and intensity of pain, relieving or aggravating factors.
- Constant, spasmodic, cramping or colicky type pain.
- Site of pain – unilateral pain may suggest pathology within the adnexae, appendicitis or ureteric colic while bilateral pain may suggest a uterine origin involving both tubes, such as endometritis and salpingitis. Suprapubic pain may indicate cystitis.

Associated symptoms

- Vaginal bleeding, vaginal discharge
- Urinary symptoms – dysuria, frequency
- Gastrointestinal and/or bowel symptoms – anorexia, vomiting, constipation, diarrhoea
- Fever

Gynaecological history

- Regular/irregular menstrual cycle
- Contraception – particularly intrauterine device (IUD) because of increased risk of ectopic pregnancy and pelvic infection
- Previous history of pelvic infections (PID)
- Previous ectopic pregnancy
- Previous history of endometriosis, infertility, fibroids
- Previous pelvic surgery, such as removal of ovarian cysts, oophorectomy, myomectomy, tubal surgery (including sterilization)
- Cervical smear history

Obstetric history
- Parity
- Previous miscarriages

Medical history
- Sickle cell disease (relevant in certain ethnic groups)
- Any other abdominal surgery – may cause adhesion leading to pain, intestinal obstruction

Review of systems
- Gastrointestinal
- Urinary

What other important aspect of this young woman's history are you particularly interested in?
Sexual history
- Previous sexual transmitted infections
- Recent sexual activity
- Change of sexual partner
- Unprotected sex

Kenzi tells you that the pain is severe, constant and she occasionally feels nauseous. She cannot remember when her last menstrual period was, but is adamant that she is not pregnant as her partner always uses condoms. She does not have any vaginal bleeding or discharge and has had no previous gynaecological surgery. She recalls that she has had a pelvic infection in the past, possibly Chlamydia, for which she and her partner were treated. She is still with the same partner.

What would you look for on physical examination?
General examination
- Body mass index
- Pallor, tachycardia and hypotensive (she could be septicaemic)
- Fever

Observation is very important. A patient with peritonitis or peritonism may be lying very still and be reluctant to move.

Abdominal examination
- Tenderness in the iliac fossae, rebound tenderness or involuntary guarding
- Suprapubic tenderness
- Her abdomen may be distended (intestinal obstruction)
- Any palpable masses

Pelvic examination
Speculum examination
The cervix should always be visualized with a Cusco speculum. A high vaginal swab should be performed as well as an endocervical swab for *Chlamydia*. Look especially for profuse yellow malodorous discharge which may indicate gonococcal or chlamydial infection. If she is pregnant, the cervical os should be inspected to determine if open or closed, or blood or products of conception observed in the vagina or in the cervical canal.

Bimanual examination
Assess the size of uterus and direction (anteverted or retroverted). An enlarged uterine size may suggest pregnancy or fibroids. Also, palpate for adnexal masses. There may be cervical excitation or tenderness, and the uterine size and adnexae may be difficult to assess because of pain. The uterus may lack mobility if there is a past history of PID or endometriosis from adhesions.

To summarize your findings so far, Kenzi is a 25-year-old para 0+0 with an acute episode of pelvic pain, especially in the left lower abdomen. She has a history of pelvic infection, possibly Chlamydia, in the past and is unsure of her last menstrual period. Her abdomen was tender on examination with guarding especially on the left side, and on speculum examination, there was a small amount of white vaginal discharge noted. It was quite difficult to assess the uterus and adnexae on bimanual examination, as they were tender.

What do you do next?
A urine pregnancy test is mandatory. This should be performed on admission to the gynaecology ward for most emergency admissions. The result of the test will influence your differential diagnosis as well as the investigations you may choose to do.

What other investigations would you recommend?
- *Full blood count.* A raised white cell count (leucocytosis) and neutrophils may suggest an inflammatory process, such as PID, ovarian torsion or appendicitis, although a normal white cell count does not exclude PID. A raised platelet count may indicate sepsis.
- *Clotting.* May be deranged in septicaemia, or following internal haemorrhage.
- *Urea and electrolytes.* May be deranged in septicaemia.

Box 2.1 Acute pelvic inflammatory disease

Pelvic inflammatory disease (PID) is usually the result of ascending infection from the endocervix causing: endometritis, salpingitis, parametritis, oophoritis, tubo-ovarian abscess and pelvic peritonitis

It can be caused by:
- *Chlamydia trachomatis*
- *Neisseria gonorrhoeae*
- *Mycoplasma genitalium*
- Anaerobes and other organisms

Clinical features
- Lower abdominal pain/tenderness
- Abnormal vaginal/cervical discharge
- Deep dyspareunia

- Fever
- Cervical excitation and adnexal tenderness

Treatment options
- Oral doxycycline and metronidazole
- Oral ofloxacin
- IM ceftriaxone or cefoxitin
- IV cefoxitin or clindamycin

Points to note
- When PID is suspected, screen for *Chlamydia* and gonorrhoea
- Sexual partners should be contacted and offered screening and treatment
- Long-term sequelae – ectopic pregnancy, infertililty, chronic pelvic pain

---

- *Group/save or group/cross-match.* Particularly in suspected ectopic pregnancy.
- *C-reactive protein (CRP).* Can indicate inflammation. This is a delayed marker and may indicate acute or chronic inflammation.
- *Sickledex/blood film.* To test for sickle cell disease.
- *Urinalysis.* Mid-stream specimen of urine (MSSU) for culture and sensitivity. Urine can also be tested for *Chlamydia* using amplification techniques.
- Endocervical and vaginal swabs.

The urine pregnancy test is negative and initial results of blood investigations for Kenzi indicate a raised white blood cell count of 17×10^9/L. In light of her pelvic pain, white vaginal discharge, leucocytosis and past history of pelvic infection you are inclined to think that she has PID and therefore commence her on antibiotics and analgesics (Box 2.1).

About 6 hours later, you are called by one of the nurses to review Kenzi. She is doubled over and complaining of worsening pain despite analgesics. She has also had two episodes of vomiting. Her pulse is 112 beats/minute.

What would you do now?

Check all observations – pulse, blood pressure, temperature and urine output. Instigate intravenous rehydration because of the vomiting.

Re-evaluate all your differential diagnoses

- *Acute PID:* still possible and worsening or persistent symptoms may be related to abscess formation

- *Mittelschmerz and/or primary dysmenorrhoea:* unlikely with this degree of severity and not resolving with analgesics
- *Endometriosis:* no previous history
- *Ovarian cyst accident:* torsion/rupture/haemorrhage have still to be excluded and could give this clinical picture
- *Gastrointestinal causes:* still to be excluded, although appendicitis less likely as pain is left-sided
- *Urinary tract infection:* unlikely if urinalysis negative

What further investigations are warranted?
Imaging
- Pelvic ultrasound
- Abdominal X-ray – indicated if a gastrointestinal cause is considered, such as intestinal obstruction

An ultrasound scan performed shows a 7-cm left-sided ovarian cyst. The patient is very tender during the scan.

How does this now affect your diagnosis?

In light of persistent pain, clinically unwell patient, leucocytosis and ultrasound findings, you think it is likely that she may have an ovarian cyst accident.

How would you manage this?
- Inform senior staff and anaesthetists
- Patient to be booked in emergency theatre for a diagnostic laparoscopy
- Keep fasted

Box 2.2 Ovarian cyst accidents

- Rupture
- Torsion
- Haemorrhage into cyst

Points to note
- Ovarian cysts can be physiological, benign or malignant
- Cysts presenting acutely are usually benign or physiological
- If complex or solid features of cyst on ultrasound, consider a serum CA125 test

Complications
- Rupture can lead to heavy blood loss
- Prolonged torsion leads to necrosis and loss of ovary, and may progress to sepsis
- Rarely, torsion can cause a coagulopathy

Treatment
- Depends on size and nature of cyst
- Some may be managed on an outpatient basis, with follow-up ultrasound scans if suspected to be physiological and small size (cysts <6 cm rarely undergo torsion)
- Analgesia
- Some may require further imaging – computed tomography (CT) scan or magnetic resonance imaging (MRI)
- Ultrasound-guided cyst aspiration may be appropriate for some
- Laparoscopy
- Laparotomy

- Rehydration – intravenous fluids
- Adequate analgesia – she is likely to require opioids, such as morphine

The patient subsequently underwent a diagnostic laparoscopy at which a torsion of the left-sided ovarian cyst was discovered (Box 2.2). A laparoscopic ovarian cystectomy was performed. Prior to the operation, Ms Anderson was consented for this procedure as well as for an oophorectomy if this was thought to be necessary, for instance in the case of a necrotic ovary, or unable to identify normal ovarian tissue within the torted mass.

What other issues would you discuss when you consent a patient for a laparoscopic procedure?

You must inform women of the risk of inadvertent trauma to major blood vessels, bowel and bladder as well as the possible need for laparotomy.

CASE REVIEW

This young woman presented with an episode of acute pelvic pain. As ectopic pregnancy is an important differential diagnosis, it is crucial that a pregnancy test be performed early on, particularly if there is a history of a missed period.

Following the history and examination findings, the initial impression in this case was an acute pelvic infection which can present with severe abdominal pain as well as findings in keeping with an acute abdomen. However, with worsening of the patient's condition, an ultrasound scan was performed which showed a large ovarian cyst. Therefore, it can be recommended that imaging be performed as part of the first line investigations for a woman with acute abdominal pain.

Ovarian cyst accidents such as rupture or haemorrhage into a cyst can be managed with analgesia and intravenous fluids if dehydrated, while a suspected torsion should have

surgical exploration. In this patient, ongoing abdominal pain, raised white blood cell count (leucocytosis), tachycardia and the discovery of an ovarian cystic mass on ultrasound scan all pointed to the diagnosis of torsion. Rapid intervention is required as prolonged torsion will compromise the blood supply to the ovary and an oophorectomy will then be required.

The benefits of laparoscopic surgery include quick recovery, less blood loss and a reduced thrombotic risk when compared with open surgery. However, there are risks of bowel and major vascular injury during any laparoscopic procedure and this may lead to a laparotomy. The patient must be advised of this and, in addition, an open procedure may be necessary in the event that the laparoscopic procedure cannot be performed, as in the presence of multiple adhesions from previous surgery or difficult access because of severe endometriosis.

KEY POINTS

- Ectopic pregnancy is an important differential diagnosis in a young woman with acute pelvic pain
- Pelvic infection can present as an acute abdomen
- A full gynaecological history, including a sexual history, is essential in assessing acute pelvic pain
- An ultrasound scan should be performed as a first line investigation in the management of pelvic pain
- *Chlamydia* is a common cause of acute PID, and recurrent infections may affect fertility and increase the risk of ectopic pregnancy
- Acute pelvic pain can be caused by non-gynaecological causes, such as appendicitis or nephrolithiasis

Case 3   A 23-year-old woman admitted as an emergency with acute vulval pain

Chloë White is 23 years old and presents with rapid onset of vulva pain. She was aware of some discomfort and tenderness the previous 2 days and noticed a swelling on the left side of her vulva when in the shower. The pain is now unbearable. She has taken paracetamol with no noticeable relief. At first she hoped it would settle on its own. She was embarrassed to be seen but now she cannot sit because the swelling is so tender.

What differential diagnoses immediately comes to mind?

- Bartholin's abscess
- Vulva abscess
- Genital herpes
- Vulva haematoma
- Behçet's disease
- Thrush infection
- Contact dermatitis

What would you like to elicit from the history?

With this presentation of acute pain, you need to make a provisional diagnosis. History-taking will allow you to develop a rapport with the patient before your examination. Examination will be revealing, help direct any further detailed questions and, importantly, allow you to make a provisional diagnosis so you can instigate pain relief.

You need to consider sexually transmitted infection (STI) but, in your initial history, you do not need to take a full sexual history. You should ask about recent sexual contact, use of contraception, previous episodes of vulva pain or discharge. You also need to clarify if she has taken any medications and if these preceded the development of her symptoms. You should ask about any possible topical irritants including washing and sanitary products and clothing. You should ask about any possible trauma. If she has been assaulted, she may not offer this information initially. With a primary herpes infection, she may have generalized symptoms of malaise, myalgia, headache and fever.

Chloë tells you that she has one regular sexual partner and has a contraceptive implant for the last 2 years. She does not use any barrier methods. She has no history of thrush or STIs. The only medication that she has taken is paracetamol since the pain started. She has very light periods with the implant but her last menstrual period (LMP) was 3 weeks previously and she has not used any sanitary products. She uses a shower gel and wears cotton 'boy shorts' type underwear.

What would you look for on physical examination?
General examination

There may be little or nothing to find on general examination. She is unlikely to have any systemic signs of infection. If you were considering a drug eruption or Behçet's disease, you need to check her oral mucosa for signs of ulceration. If she has a Bartholin's abscess or herpes infection, she may have inguinal lymphadenopathy.

Pelvic examination

You need to make a visual inspection of her vulva but you must explain exactly what you intend to do as she is in considerable pain. It may not be possible to do more than an inspection so make sure that you have an adequate light source as this should lead you to the diagnosis. There is no indication to do an internal examination at this stage and she would be unable to tolerate this procedure.

Obstetrics and Gynaecology: Clinical Cases Uncovered.
By M. Cruickshank and A. Shetty. Published 2009 by Blackwell Publishing. ISBN 978-1-4051-8671-1.

Box 3.1 Bartholin's gland

There are two Bartholin's glands situated on either side of the posterior fourchette. The duct from each gland drains into the lower vagina between the hymenal remnants (carunculae myrtiformes) and the fourchette. Blockage of the gland can result in a mucous retention cyst which can grow to 3–5 cm in diameter and presents as a vuval swelling. Infection results in an abscess which presents with pain. This is seen more often than a cyst.

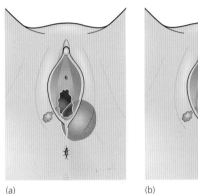 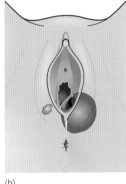

(a)   (b)

Figure 3.1 (a) Site of Bartholin's gland and duct and (b) marsupialization of a Bartholin's abscess.

To summarize your findings so far, Chloë is a 23-year-old para 0+0 with 48-hour history of increasing vulva swelling associated tenderness and pain. On examination, she has an erythematous tender swelling localized to the left side of her posterior fourchette. The swelling has surrounding induration and she has a tender lymphadenopathy in her left inguinal region.

What do you do next?

You do not need to obtain any further investigations at this stage. She has a Bartholin's abscess and you should assess her for an anaesthetic and book her for emergency surgery (Box 3.1; Fig. 3.1 and Fig. 3.2).

What surgical procedure is necessary?
Marsupialization of Bartholin's abscess

The underlying pathology is blockage of the duct draining from the Bartholin's gland. Simple incision and drainage will not allow the duct to drain so marsupialization is performed. An ellipse of overlying vaginal mucous is excised along with the abscess wall to allow the pus to drain. The edges are sewn together with an interrupted

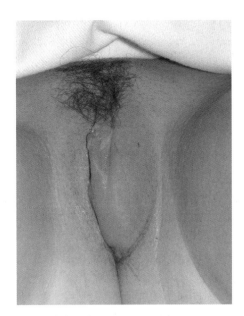

Figure 3.2 Bartholin's abcess.

dissolvable suture to maintain patency. Postoperatively this will reduce to a tiny opening.

Now review your differential diagnosis
Vulva abscess

Although your examination findings confirm an abscess, the anatomical site clinches the diagnosis. A vulval abscess is more likely to be found in the hair-bearing skin of the labia majora or mons pubis arising in hair follicles, sweat glands or sebaceous glands. Anyone can develop a skin abscess but this can be associated with diabetes. These are treated by incision and drainage. In hydradenitis suppurativa, a disorder of the sweat glands, multiple small abscesses and scarring are found in the anogenital and axillary areas. This often starts in teenagers or young adults and is more common in women.

Herpes virus infection

A primary herpes virus infection (HSV) can be extremely painful and require hospital admission. The pain is bilateral and generalized. Chloë does not have risk factors for HSV (number of sexual partners or previous history of STIs) although she does not use barrier contraception. Genital herpes usually presents 2–14 days after sexual contact. Admission may be necessary in the case of secondary urinary retention requiring catheterization.

On examination, you would expect to see multiple papules, vesicles or shallow ulcers with associated erythema, oedema and crusting. A swab should be taken to confirm the diagnosis and allow counselling on future recurrence. However, if you suspect herpes you should start antiviral therapy immediately with aciclovir 400 mg three times per day for 7–10 days for an primary episode. If she is in acute urinary retention, she will have severe lower abdominal pain and a tender distended bladder will be palpable on abdominal examination. This complication may be caused by inhibition secondary to pain, local swelling or neuropathic from nerve root involvement. You may have to insert a suprapubic catheter. Topical anaesthetic gel can be useful for pain relief. You need to arrange follow-up at genitourinary medicine (GUM) clinic to screen for other STIs.

Vulva haematoma

Haematoma is related to trauma and is seen more commonly following childbirth but it is also seen following accidental injury (e.g. straddle injury) or non-accidental injury where internal penetrative injuries to other structures (e.g. bladder, bowel and vagina) need to be excluded. It is also a complication of vaginal surgery if a haematoma forms below the level of the pelvic floor and blood tracks down the loose tissue planes into the vulva and buttock. Haematomas cause a tender swelling and the blood causes discoloration which is obvious in association with a history of trauma.

Haematomas are self-limiting and can be managed conservatively with pain relief, catheterization and blood transfusion if necessary. If large, you may consider exploration and drainage. As bleeding is often from the venous plexus rather than arterial, no obvious bleeding points may be found after evacuation of haematoma and you may need to leave in a drain to avoid reaccumulation. Trauma above the level of the pelvic floor (pelvic or vaginal surgery, childbirth or penetrating injury) will not track down to the vulva so there are no external findings.

Behçet's disease

This is a chronic autoimmune disorder with recurrent episodes of mouth ulcers. It can be associated with vulva ulceration. Autoimmune disorders tend to present for the first time in young women and this condition is more common in women presenting for the first time aged 20–40 years. There is no diagnostic test and other conditions, especially herpes, need to be excluded. A fixed drug eruption can present with a similar appearance of vulva redness and swelling and blistering which is extremely painful. It starts within minutes or hours of taking the precipitating medication and can be caused by paracetamol or ibuprofen. Chloë gives no preceding history of drug-taking or previous episodes of mouth ulcers.

Thrush infection

Vulva candidiasis can cause inflammation, excoriation and pain as well as itch. However, it does not develop rapidly as in this case nor be severe enough to require admission. On examination, there may be bilateral erythema and inflammation with a leading edge or satellite lesions. This can require a prolonged course of topical antifungal therapy to clear.

Contact dermatitis

Chloë gives no obvious history of contact irritants. Swelling and erythema would be bilateral involving the area in contact with the sensitizer. Dermatitis is more likely to cause itch with pain secondary to irritation and itching damaging the skin.

On recovery from her anaesthetic, Chloë feels much better and is able to be discharged later the same day. A swab taken from the abscess in theatre grows mixed anaerobes. Antibiotics are only required if there is an associated cellulitis. She may develop another Bartholin's abscess in the future but the recurrence rate is low so no follow-up is required.

CASE REVIEW

Women with severe vulva pain may be admitted as an emergency to the gynaecology ward. Occasionally, this is caused by uncommon dermatological conditions (Behçet's disease, fixed drug eruption, pemphigus) and liaison with the dermatology department is essential.

However, there are a few common gynaecological causes for this symptom. Bartholin's abscess is often seen but may also be referred to the outpatient clinic as a Bartholin's cyst. The diagnosis is obvious on clinical examination because of its anatomical location. Pain relief will be obtained by draining the abscess so theatre needs to be booked. While waiting to go to theatre, you should provide adequate analgesia and a hot bath may help. It is necessary to marsupialize the abscess rather than simple incision and drainage which has a higher risk of recurrence as the gland duct remains blocked. The usual causal organisms are mixed anaerobes, but occasionally there can be a specific organism such as gonorrhoea or chlamydia so a swab should be taken from the abscess in theatre.

In this age group, a primary HSV infection is likely and may be associated with considerable erythema and oedema. However, this will be generalized and bilateral. It may result in urinary retention and you may need to use a suprapubic catheter to relieve the retention. There may also be systemic symptoms of malaise, fever and myalgia. Recurrence is common but future attacks tend to be less severe and aciclovir should be taken as soon as any prodromal symptoms are experienced to lessen the severity and duration of the attack.

Vulva haematoma will be obvious on examination. There will be a history of a straddle type injury with bleeding arising from the rich venous plexus of the vulva or a penetrating injury to the vagina with tracking of blood downwards. With vaginal lacerations, you will need to examine the patient under anaesthetic to identify any injury to bladder, bowel or perforation of the peritoneum and suture any vaginal lacerations. If there is no clear history of trauma, you need to consider non-accidental injury.

KEY POINTS

- Acute vulva pain is a common emergency admission to the gynaecology department
- Women are often in considerable pain so you need to provide analgesia promptly
- The diagnosis can usually be made on inspection and your examination may be limited to this aspect only if the woman is in pain
- Bartholin's abscess is common and is diagnosed by the anatomical site of the abscess

- Bartholin's abscess requires marsupialization to allow the gland to drain and reduce the risk of recurrence
- If you suspect HSV, you need to instigate management before you have swab results available
- If HSV is confirmed, you need to arrange follow-up at GUM for counselling and a full STI screen
- Vulva haematomas can often be managed conservatively but exploration is required if they are increasing in size or if they result from a penetrating injury

Case 4 A 45-year-old woman with heavy periods

Mrs Ellen Smith is a 45-year-old woman who presents with heavy periods. This started about 8 months ago and the bleeding has become increasingly heavy. She is now quite distressed about this problem.

What differential diagnoses immediately come to mind?

- Dysfunctional uterine bleeding (DUB)
- Uterine fibroids
- Endometrial polyp
- Endometrial hyperplasia
- Endometriosis
- Adenomyosis
- Endometrial cancer

What would you like to elicit from the history?

Presenting complaint and history of presenting complaint

- Frequency and duration of vaginal bleeding
- Intermenstrual or postcoital bleeding
- Associated pain

Associated symptoms

- Symptoms of anaemia: lethargy, fatigue, palpitations

Menstrual history

- Duration, frequency and regularity of menses prior to this problem
- Age of menarche
- Contraception, in particular intrauterine device (IUD) or hormone replacement therapy (HRT)
- Cervical smear history, particularly date and result of last smear test

Obstetric history

- Parity, type of deliveries, any complications

Medical history

- Thyroid disease, hypertension, diabetes
- Bleeding or clotting disorders

Family history

- History of cancer, particularly endometrial, colon, breast
- Bleeding or clotting disorders

What aspects of this woman's social history are you particularly interested in?

Heavy menstrual bleeding has a major impact on a woman's quality of life, and this can help in quantifying the amount of vaginal loss. For instance, having to take time off work because the bleeding is too heavy, not wanting to leave the house for fear of an 'accident' or not going on holiday because of the inconvenience of bleeding will give an indication of the effect this problem has on the patient's life.

The National Institute for Clinical Excellence (NICE) defines heavy menstrual bleeding as excessive menstrual blood loss that interferes with the woman's physical, emotional, social and material quality of life. It is therefore not only useful to enquire about her job, smoking or alcohol status, but to assess how much this problem is affecting her day-to-day activities.

Mrs Smith tells you that her periods are lasting longer and it is sometimes difficult to tell what is her period or bleeding in between her periods (intermenstrual bleeding). This haphazard pattern is causing her great distress as she feels she cannot continue with her outdoor lifestyle which includes cycling.

Obstetrics and Gynaecology: Clinical Cases Uncovered.
By M. Cruickshank and A. Shetty. Published 2009 by Blackwell Publishing. ISBN 978-1-4051-8671-1.

What would you look for on physical examination?

General examination
- Body mass index (BMI)
- Pallor and tachycardia may indicate anaemia
- Remember to check mucous membranes for pallor in dark women

Abdominal examination
This may be completely normal. A pelvic mass may be palpable in the case of a fibroid uterus. The size of a mass arising from the pelvis is measured and stated relative to a pregnant uterus, e.g. a mass felt up to the level of the umbilicus is 20–22 weeks size.

Pelvic examination

Speculum examination
The cervix should always be visualized with a Cusco speculum. Look for polyps or ectopy. A cervix clinically suspicious of cancer should be referred for an urgent opinion. You only need to take a vaginal or endocervical swab if infection is suspected.

Bimanual examination
You need to assess the size of the uterus relative to that of a pregnant uterus and whether it is anteverted or retroverted. Feel on either side for adnexal masses. An enlarged uterus may suggest fibroids or adenomyosis.

> To summarize your findings so far, Mrs Smith is a 45-year-old para 2+0 (both caesarean sections) with an 8-month history of irregular heavy menstrual bleeding which is now affecting her quality of life. She is up to date with cervical smears, and has no past medical history of note. On examination, her BMI is 35, and there were no obvious abnormal findings, although it is appreciated that it was difficult to assess the abdomen and pelvis because of her size.

What do you do next?
1 An *endometrial biopsy* should be taken. Although endometrial cancer is uncommon in women under 40 years, the incidence rises between 40 and 55 years. Risk factors include obesity, polycystic ovarian syndrome (PCOS), nulliparity, unopposed oestrogen replacement therapy, tamoxifen and feminizing ovarian tumours such as thecomas or granulosa cell tumours.

Box 4.1 Uterine fibroids (leiomyomas)

- Most common benign tumour of the female genital tract
- Found particularly in black/African/Afro-Caribbean women
- Oestrogen-dependent
- Can be intramural, subserosal, submucosal or pedunculated

The indications for taking an endometrial biopsy in women with menorrhagia are:
- age 45 years and above
- persistent intermenstrual bleeding
- treatment failure

An endometrial biopsy is a safe and simple procedure which is usually well-tolerated as an outpatient procedure and should be performed at this first visit.

2 *Full blood count* (FBC) to check for iron deficiency anaemia secondary to blood loss.

3 *Pelvic ultrasound scan*. This will identify structural abnormalities and detect endometrial polyps, uterine fibroids and uterine malformations (Box 4.1). It may show unusual appearances suggestive of malignancy.

> However, an ultrasound performed showed a slightly bulky uterus, no fibroids and no endometrial polyps. Both ovaries appeared normal. An FBC reports a haemoglobin level at the lower limit of normal at 110 g/L. You had difficulty performing a Pipelle endometrial biopsy, which is common when a woman has not had any vaginal deliveries, as in this case.

What would you do next?
If available, an outpatient hysteroscopy may be attempted under local anaesthetic. Alternatively, a diagnostic hysteroscopy can be performed in theatre under a general anaesthetic. This should be carried out as an inpatient with an anaesthetic assessment for this patient because of her high BMI. A hysteroscopy is the gold standard for evaluating the uterine cavity and could show endometrial polyps, submucosal fibroids, fibroid polyps, as well as endometrial cancer and can allow a biopsy to be taken. A dilatation and curettage is no longer a recommended investigation as pathology may be missed without inspection of the uterine cavity.

> Following the results of all investigations, including a diagnostic hysteroscopy, there are no significant

---

Box 4.2 Dysfunctional uterine bleeding

- DUB is a very common cause of abnormal vaginal bleeding
- This diagnosis should only be made after ruling out organic and structural causes for abnormal vaginal bleeding
- About 90% of DUB results from anovulation and 10% occurs with ovulatory cycles
- During an anovulatory cycle, the corpus luteum fails to form, which causes failure of normal cyclical progesterone secretion
- This results in continuous unopposed production of oestradiol, stimulating overgrowth of the endometrium. Without progesterone, the endometrium proliferates and eventually outgrows its blood supply, leading to necrosis. The end result is overproduction of uterine blood flow
- In ovulatory DUB, prolonged progesterone secretion causes irregular shedding of the endometrium
- DUB is common at the extremes of a woman's reproductive years. In this patient, who may be peri-menopausal, DUB could be an early manifestation of ovarian failure

---

Box 4.3 Adenomyosis

- Adenomyosis is the presence of endometrial tissue within the muscle of the uterus (myometrium) where it is not normally found
- When the endometrial tissue grows during the menstrual cycle and then at menses tries to slough off, the old tissue and blood cannot escape the uterine muscle and flow out of the cervix as part of normal menses. This trapping of the blood and tissue causes uterine pain in the form of monthly menstrual cramps (dysmenorrhoea)
- It also produces abnormal uterine bleeding when some of the blood finally escapes the muscle, resulting in prolonged spotting
- The uterus is uniform in outline and may be minimally enlarged
- Adenomyosis is difficult to diagnose and is usually only detected on histopathological examination of the uterus following hysterectomy

---

structural abnormalities detected and an endometrial biopsy shows no hyperplasia, atypia or malignancy.

Now, review all your differential diagnoses

- *Uterine fibroids:* none seen on ultrasound scan or hysteroscopy, so unlikely
- *Dysfunctional uterine bleeding:* most likely cause so far as no structural abnormality detected (Box 4.2)
- *Endometrial polyp:* although initially plausible, none seen on ultrasound scan or hysteroscopy, so unlikely
- *Endometrial hyperplasia:* not detected on biopsy of endometrium
- *Endometriosis:* somewhat unlikely in this age group and usually accompanied with pelvic pain and dysmenorrhoea
- *Adenomyosis:* possible as bulky uterus noted on ultrasound scan, but cannot be definitively diagnosed other than histopathological examination of the uterus following hysterectomy (Box 4.3)
- *Endometrial cancer:* not detected on biopsy of endometrium

What treatment options would you offer this patient?

It is important to note that any intervention should aim to improve the woman's quality of life rather than focusing on menstrual blood loss. NICE recommends that treatment and care should take into account the woman's needs and preferences and good communication is essential in allowing women to make informed decisions about their care (Tables 4.1 & 4.2).

At a subsequent visit, you suggest the option of a Mirena coil to Mrs Smith, but she does not seem to be keen as she has had a coil in the past, but 'it did not agree with her'. You explain that unlike other contraceptive IUDs, this is an intrauterine system (IUS) which works differently and may improve her symptoms. However, she would prefer not to try it and, following further detailed discussion, a microwave endometrial ablation (MEA) is chosen. She seems happy about this option.

Three months following the MEA, you review Mrs Smith. She is much happier with the vaginal bleeding, which she says is very much reduced. She does complain of occasional cramping abdominal pain, but can otherwise continue with her active lifestyle.

Table 4.1 Medical (pharmaceutical) treatment.

Treatment	How does it work	Side-effects
LNG-IUS, Mirena	A hormonal intrauterine device that slowly releases progestogen and prevents proliferation of the endometrium. It also thickens the cervical mucus and acts as a contraceptive	Irregular spotting, bleeding for first 3–6 months. Breast tenderness, acne, headaches. Small risk of uterine perforation at insertion Not useful with large fibroids distorting the uterine cavity
Tranexamic acid	A non-hormonal oral antifibrinolytic	Uncommon side-effects, occasionally indigestion, headache
NSAIDs	Reduce prostaglandin production	Indigestion, diarrhoea. Not for use with peptic ulcer disease
Combined oral contraceptive	Stops ovulation, prevents proliferation of endometrium	Breast tenderness, nausea, mood changes. Rarely, deep vein thrombosis. Therefore not for use in those with past history of thrombotic events
GnRH analogues	Monthly injection that stops oestrogen and progesterone production	Causes menopausal-like symptoms such as hot flushes, night sweats and vaginal dryness
	A temporary measure to shrink fibroids prior to surgery, or to 'buy time' if peri-menopausal	Cannot be used for more than 6 months, as can be associated with osteoporosis

GnRH, gonadotrophin releasing hormone; LNG-IUS, levonorgestrel-releasing intrauterine system; NSAID, non-steroidal anti-inflammatory drug.

CASE REVIEW

This woman presented with heavy menstrual bleeding, one of the most common gynaecological complaints. It is important to assess the quantity of menstrual blood loss particularly in relation to how this influences her daily life.

There were no obvious abnormalities detected on examination and investigations including an ultrasound scan and hysteroscopy similarly were negative. Heavy menstrual bleeding can be caused by DUB which occurs in the absence of structural abnormalities. However, it is recommended that an endometrial biopsy is performed in women over the age of 40 years who complain of any change in menstrual pattern. This should also be performed prior to any form of endometrial ablation. Obesity, as well as the inability to perform a Pipelle sample in this case, provided an additional challenge which may be frequently encountered.

All treatment options, both medical and surgical, should be fully discussed with the patient and a decision made depending on expected results and possible side-effects. In this case, medical therapy may not have been the best selection, while a hysterectomy can be considered to be extreme as the first option for treatment. Hysterectomy is the most invasive form of treatment and risks such as haemorrhage, thrombosis and infection are greater than for less invasive techniques such as the Mirena IUS or endometrial ablation. However, it is essential that women are aware that endometrial ablation can reduce menstrual loss, but may not cause amenorrhoea.

Table 4.2 Surgical and radiological treatment.

Treatment	How does it work	Side-effects
Endometrial ablation for women with: • normal or small uterus (<10 weeks) • no desire to conceive • only small fibroids (<3 cm diameter)	Destroys endometrium using: • microwave • balloon thermal • radiofrequency • roller ball • transcervical resection	• Vaginal discharge, pelvic pain, infection, uncommonly perforation • Does not cause amenorrhoea, may need additional surgery
Hysteroscopic resection of fibroid for women with: • submucosal fibroid/fibroid polyp • fibroid size >3 cm • desire to conceive	Surgical removal of fibroids using a hysteroscope	• Infection, intrauterine adhesions which may affect fertility, haemorrhage, perforation, recurrence of fibroids
Uterine artery embolization for women who: • want to retain uterus • want to avoid surgery • have fibroids >3 cm	Cuts off blood supply to the fibroids by injecting small particles in the blood vessels supplying the uterus	• Vaginal discharge, post-embolization syndrome (pain, fever, vomiting) • May need additional surgery • Premature ovarian failure, especially >45 years old • Rarely, haemorrhage, septicaemia
Myomectomy for women who: • have large fibroids • want to retain fertility	Surgical removal of fibroids	• Adhesions, may affect fertility, may need additional surgery, fibroid recurrence, infection
Hysterectomy: • not first-line • when other treatment have failed • no desire to retain fertility or uterus	Surgical removal of uterus (ovaries can also be removed if appropriate). Can be: • vaginal • abdominal • LAVH – particularly useful in obese women	• Intra- or postoperative haemorrhage, infection (UTI, wound), damage to other structures, such as bowel or bladder at operation; rarely, deep vein thrombosis, pulmonary embolus

LAVH, laparoscopic-assisted vaginal hysterectomy; UTI, urinary tract infection.

KEY POINTS

• Heavy menstrual bleeding can affect a woman's lifestyle, and the extent that this is affected will help in selecting the best form of treatment
• Diagnostic investigations include ultrasound scan, endometrial biopsy and hysteroscopy
• Uterine fibroids can cause menorrhagia, and treatment may depend on the patient's fertility status

• Adenomyosis can only be confirmed on histopathological review of a hysterectomy specimen
• DUB is usually the cause of heavy menstrual bleeding once structural or organic causes are excluded
• Medical or surgical therapy is recommended depending on the diagnosis and patients should be counselled on all viable options

A 52-year-old woman who has not been able to control her temper recently

Mrs Caroline Britain, a 52-year-old business executive, has noticed that over the last few months she has not been able to control her temper in difficult meetings and becomes red and flustered. This has become both embarrassing for potential clients and senior management. Her secretary who has worked for her for over 10 years has heard gossip around the office. She feels she has to broach the subject when Mrs Britain walks out of a very important meeting for the company after shouting at a client. Mrs Britain receives a verbal warning because of her actions. After Mrs Britain discusses this distressing event with her secretary, she attends her GP. She admits to marital problems secondary to difficulties with sex and sleeping because of sweating.

What is your differential diagnosis?
* Anxiety/depression
* Menopausal symptoms
* Thyroid dysfunction

What do you need to elicit from the history?
History of complaint
* Presence of hot flushes/night sweats and subsequent requirements, e.g. showering overnight, changing night wear or bed clothes
* Duration of symptoms
* Amenorrhoea or irregular/less frequent periods
* Vaginal bleeding or discharge
* Presence of palpitations, anxiety, diarrhoea
* Difficulty in getting to sleep or waking at night and unable to get back to sleep

* Extent of marital difficulties including sexual issues such as dysparunia, aparunia

Associated symptoms
* *Urinary symptoms:* frequency or dysuria
* *Bowel symptoms:* diarrhoea and abdominal pain

Menstrual history
* Last menstrual period (LMP) and regularity of periods

Screening history
* Mammogram result
* Smear history
* Presence of significant venous varicosities in lower limbs

Obstetric history
* Parity, type of delivery and complications

Medical history
Any previous history of hypertension, osteoporosis, ischaemic heart disease, strokes, hysterectomy, gynaecological malignancy, previous endometriosis, previous/present breast cancer, thrombotic episodes (e.g. pulmonary embolism, deep venous thrombosis).

Family history
Ask about the presence of hypertension, ischaemic heart disease, osteoporosis, thyroid dysfunction, breast/gynaecological cancer and thrombotic episodes.

Drug history
Ask about non-prescribed and prescribed medication.

Mrs Britain explains her LMP was 10 months ago and since then she has had difficulty sleeping because of hot flushes and night sweats. Sometimes she has to shower three or four times a night to cool down. This has led to marital difficulties because of the constant

Obstetrics and Gynaecology: Clinical Cases Uncovered.
By M. Cruickshank and A. Shetty. Published 2009 by Blackwell Publishing. ISBN 978-1-4051-8671-1.

disruption of getting up at night and her reduced libido. She finds intercourse is painful and can precipitate the hot flushes and sweats. The lack of sleep has caused her difficulty to cope at work.

She has two grown-up children; both delivered uneventfully and she has never had any gynaecological operations. Both her smears and mammograms are up to date and have been normal. She has noticed some urinary frequency and 'stinging', but it is intermittent and no urinary infection has been identified from culture despite several samples being tested. Mrs Britain does admit that this mainly occurs after trying to have intercourse which is painful on entry and during intercourse. She has found it less painful with a lubricant that she bought over-the-counter. The night sweats are the main problem affecting her quality of life as she cannot function properly during the day because they disturb her sleep pattern. She did try some homeopathic preparation from the local health shop, but it did not work, so she stopped taking it 3 months ago.

What would you look for on physical examination?
General examination
- Tired appearance
- Presence of flushing/sweating during consultation
- Presence of goitre

Vaginal examination

First you need to look for the presence of atrophic change. There may be petechial haemorrhages around the vulva, inside the vagina or on the cervix. These may cause bleeding during the examination and you need to inform her that this is present. Sometimes the presence of petechial haemorrhage only occurs with the examination (even though you are being gentle) and indicates atrophy. If she has had previous vaginal bleeding, a transvaginal ultrasound scan to assess endometrial thickness and possible endometrial biopsy may be required. A bimanual pelvic examination should be performed if possible to exclude any enlargement of the pelvic organs or indeed pain on palpation in case dual pathology is present. The use of a lubricant and an appropriately sized speculum is important given the presence of dysparunia. In addition, remember your communication skills during the procedure and ensure that Mrs Britain can stop the examination if she finds it too painful.

To summarize your findings so far, Mrs Britain, a 52-year-old woman with 10 months of amenorrhoea, has been experiencing hot flushes and night sweats. These have impacted on both her personal and working life. She has dysparunia which has caused sexual problems with her husband, negatively affecting her mood.

On examination, Mrs Britain appeared tired, has no goitre and experienced several noticeable flushes throughout the 15-minute consultation. She does have atrophic changes within the vagina, but no provoked bleeding on examination. There are no pelvic masses and her uterus is normal sized and mobile. The main discomfort was found on insertion of the speculum, even with sufficient lubricant.

What do you do next?
General and female health screening

First, both general and female health screening are required if these have not taken place previously. Blood pressure measurements are taken especially for those who have a raised body mass index (BMI), treated hypertension or have a family history of hypertension or vascular disease. In addition to encouragement to participate in general female population screening procedures such as cervical smears or mammograms, it may be appropriate to teach the patient breast awareness (regular self-examination). Any hormone replacement that is commenced can reduce the clarity of identifying any discrete tumours so prior mammographic screening and examination is beneficial for those over 50 years if this has not been performed.

Do you need to do any investigations?

Serum samples such as follicle stimulating hormone (FSH) are not always necessary for diagnosis of the menopause. A raised FSH level (>35 IU/L) does not necessarily provide confirmation of menopause as women who are perimenopausal can have fluctuating levels dependent on the ovarian activity at the time of the blood sample being taken. To clarify the diagnosis it can be useful to perform a series of FSH levels in combination with oestradiol levels. If the oestradiol level is consistently low (<0.11 nmol/L) this is more indicative of failing activity of the ovaries as FSH levels can be erratic and wide ranging in the perimenopause.

Although not always necessary, thyroid function screening could be considered as thyroid dysfunction can occur at the perimenopause and diagnosis is hindered by menopausal symptoms. This investigation will be dictated by history and examination (especially of the thyroid region).

> You can now review your findings
> - BMI of 30
> - BP 110/75 mmHg
> - Cervical smear: normal with routine recall advised.
> - Mammogram: normal with routine recall advised.
> - FSH 90 IU/L and oestradiol less than 0.11 nmol/L
> - Normal thyroxine but raised thyroid stimulating hormone (TSH)

Now review each differential diagnosis
Anxiety/depression
Although not completely excluded as a diagnosis, the physical symptoms Mrs Britain describes are those of vasomotor symptoms and are not associated with the adrenaline/noradrenaline system.

Menopausal symptoms
This appears to be the most likely diagnosis given the raised FSH and very low oestrogen in conjunction with the present history of vasomotor symptoms and 10 months of amenorrhoea in addition to the presence of vaginal atrophy (Box 5.1).

Thyroid dysfunction
This is unlikely at present to be a cause for her presenting symptoms. However, this does require more investigation by further sampling (normally with samples 3–6 months apart) to identify any associated perimenopausal thyroid dysfunction.

Box 5.1 Effects of menopause

Short-term effects of menopause
- Hot flushes
- Night sweats
- Atrophic genitalia

Long-term effects of menopause
- Osteoporosis
- Atrophic tissues

What treatment would you offer this patient?
The use of treatments depends upon the patient, some just need advice and reassurance, others cannot cope with daily living activities (DLAs) and these are the patients who should be offered some form of treatment. The level of intrusion on DLAs will provide information on the required treatment. If the symptoms are mild, an over-the-counter preparation may be sufficient, but if symptoms are significant a more medical approach is necessary.

Herbal and homeopathic treatment
There are several preparations that are offered over-the-counter to alleviate menopausal symptoms. None of these preparations have been clinically tested other than Red Clover™ (Novogen), although this used a dose double that advised by the manufacturers. Red Clover is not yet available on NHS prescription and requires self-funding by the patient.

Many herbal preparations are known to affect intracellular activities within the body, notably co-enzyme p450, or interact with prescribed medication (such as antihypertensives, hormonal treatments, tamoxifen and antidepressants; Table 5.1). Many menopause preparations contain a combination of ingredients and patients should be made aware of the information given by the manufacturer.

Table 5.1 Warnings associated with menopausal preparations*.

Herbal preparation	Interaction/effect
St John's wort	HRT
	Antidepressants
	Contraceptive pills
	Warfarin
Kava	Liver function
	Tamoxifen
Sage	Antihypertensives

HRT, hormone replacement therapy.

* There may be several unknown at present.

Table 5.2 Types of available preparations for hormone replacement therapy.

Mode of delivery	Constituent hormones
Oral	Separate or combinations of oestrogen and/or progesterone
Transdermal	Combinations of oestrogen and progesterone or oestrogen only
Subcutaneous	Oestrogen only
	Testosterone only
Transvaginal	Oestrogen only
	Progesterone only

KEY POINT

The use of herbal preparations is at the discretion of the patient but you should guide and advise if the patient is using any prescribed medication

---

Hormone replacement therapy

There are several different hormonal preparations of HRT as well as different modes of administration (Table 5.2). The hormones required in the HRT preparation are dependent upon the patient's medical history. Oestrogens are very effective in controlling vasomotor symptoms.

KEY POINT

If the patient has had a hysterectomy only oestrogen is required.

In the case of Mrs Britain who still has a uterus, she requires both oestrogen and a progestogen.

Progesterone

The progesterone will protect and control the growth of the endometrium from the oestrogenic influence. There are two ways of giving progestogens: on a sequential or a continuous basis. The choice is dependent on the patient's duration of amenorrhoea and age. If a patient is at least 54 years old or has had at least 1 year of amenorrhoea, most patients can be given an HRT with a continuous progesto-

gen. This allows the patient to continue to experience amenorrhoea. You need to advise that there may be light intermittent bleeding in the first few months of treatment.

Mrs Britain has not had 12 months of amenorrhoea so she will need to use an HRT that contains a sequential (cyclical) progestogen and she will experience a withdrawal bleed.

KEY POINT

If she was given a continuous progestogen, she could experience very erratic and unacceptable bleeding as she will still be producing some endogenous oestrogen from her failing ovaries.

Mrs Britain has only ever taken tablets and is interested in the different routes of delivery.

There are several ways in which HRT can be given and this should be discussed with the patient and any medical problems taken into account. Different modes of delivery are beneficial for different patients. Mrs Britain has no absorption problems and could easily be offered a range of HRT delivery modes.

Transdermal preparations remove the first pass effect through the liver and are suitable for women who cannot swallow tablets or remember to take them. Women who tend to forget to take regular medication may require modes of delivery which require no thought on their part such as the implant. Vaginal preparations can be used for local vaginal symptoms. The main indicator is personal choice and the beneficial effect on her symptoms.

KEY POINT

HRT needs to be used consistently and correctly for at least 3 months before it can be considered ineffective.

Mrs Britain has no personal or family medical history to suggest any form of HRT would be better for her health, but first she wants to know about common side-effects.

What are the common side-effects of HRT?

On commencement, HRT can cause breast tenderness, slight fluid retention and skin changes, but these normally settle down over 4 months.

Mrs Britain has read a recent article about HRT and she wants to know about any risks

Counselling about the potential risks of HRT use is the most important aspect of an HRT consultation. Over the last decade, HRT use has declined because of negative media coverage of studies reported in well-respected journals. The crucial conclusions from these studies have now been amended following reanalysis of the data. The present understanding is that HRT should be used for the shortest possible time at the lowest possible dose. However, all women are individual and Mrs Britain may require HRT for several years until she can cope without it; in her case this would be her shortest possible time.

What risks should you discuss with her?

• *Breast cancer.* The main concern for women using HRT is breast cancer which increases over time in most women after the age of 50, but depends on the type of HRT used and their own family and personal history.

• *Thromboembolic disorders.* Mrs Britain, as in all patients who are considering HRT, should be informed of the slight increased risk of clotting (from 1 in 10,000 to 3 in 10,000).

• *Hypertension.* All patients should be reviewed for blood pressure checks and symptom control.

Does Mrs Britain need to have her hormone levels monitored?

She does not require further serum samples measuring FSH and oestrogen and her replacement treatment should be based on her symptoms. Some oestrogens used in HRT are not measured by the assays used on serum samples. As Mrs Britain is fit and healthy, 3-monthly BP checks are all that is required as well as symptom control.

Mrs Britain decides upon oral HRT and has no symptoms at her 3-month review apart from some residual intermittent dysparunia. On examination, the atrophic changes have improved, with no pain on speculum examination and she informs her GP she can have sex without pain.

It is decided that her GP will review her annually to identify the need for HRT continuation but provisionally a plan is agreed with her to stop the HRT at 55 years on a gradual basis. If HRT dosage reduction causes unacceptable vasomotor symptoms, then HRT will be continued and further reduction or cessation can be attempted on a yearly bases with a deadline at 60 years of age.

CASE REVIEW

This 52-year-old woman was experiencing a reduction in quality of life because of a poor sleep pattern caused by her night sweats. She found that having hot flushes caused distress at work and poor relationships were being developed both at home and work because of her physical symptoms. She had no past history and was up to date with health screening. The clinical history suggested menopausal symptoms but over-the-counter preparations had been suggested previously and tried with no success.

HRT was the most appropriate option as her symptoms were significantly affecting quality of life. On their introduction, initial screening tests were undertaken to prevent known complications of their use. She was given adequate counselling about the possible risks of using HRT. This should be directed and dependent on each individual.

KEY POINTS

• A progesterone is essential if the uterus is still in place as unopposed oestrogen significantly increases the risk of endometrial cancer
• FSH levels measurement is not necessary and a one-off level does not confirm the menopause
• Oral HRT may not be the most appropriate preparation
• A patient considering HRT should be counselled on an individual basis dependent on her family's and her own medical history

• Over-the-counter menopause preparations may not be safe for some women and a full drug history should be taken to avoid drug interactions
• Thyroid function tests can be influenced by changes in oestrogen–progesterone levels
• HRT should be used at the lowest possible dose for the shortest time on an individual basis

Case 6 A 58-year-old woman with postmenopausal bleeding

Luisa Riglinski is 58-year-old cook at a local secondary school. She thinks her last menstrual period was about 6–7 years ago. Two months ago she had a few days of vaginal bleeding which was like the end of period and since then she has continued to spot most days. This is dark red or brown and she has taken to wearing panty liners. She has no pain or any associated symptoms. Initially she thought that her periods had restarted but a friend told her that she should see her GP. She has no pain or any other symptoms. She has never been on hormone replacement therapy (HRT).

What are the most likely causes of her bleeding?

- Endometrial cancer
- Atrophic vaginitis
- Local cervical lesion
- Cervical cancer
- Iatrogenic
- *Chlamydia* infection

What further questions would help to establish the diagnosis?
History of bleeding

Postmenopausal bleeding (PMB) is defined as bleeding more than 12 months since a woman's last normal menstrual period so you need to establish when this was. You should ask about the amount and duration of bleeding and any associated symptoms. Try to clarify the site of bleeding to confirm that it is vaginal and not rectal or in her urine. Some women may find this very difficult to define.

Smear history

You need to check if she has attended for cervical screening and the result of her last smear test.

Drug history

Iatrogenic causes are important so you need to take a drug history. HRT is a common cause of PMB and if she is taking HRT, you need to ask about unscheduled bleeds; bleeding not at the time of the withdrawal bleed for women in taking a cyclical preparation or bleeding on continuous combined preparations. Check if she has had any problems with compliance, absorption (e.g. gastrointestinal upset) or metabolism (see Case 8).

Women currently or previously on tamoxifen are at increased risk of endometrial polyps, endometrial cancer and endometrial sarcoma although vaginal bleeding is a common side-effect.

Sexual history

Although *Chlamydia* infection is less common in older women, you should not ignore this as a possible cause. You do not need to take a full sexual history but you should ask if she has changed her sexual partner in the last 12 months.

KEY POINT

Women who continue to have periods after the age of 55 years also need to be investigated as for PMB.

Mrs Riglinski tells you that she has never been on HRT or tamoxifen (Box 6.1). She has no history of breast cancer. She had regular smears with normal results until the age of 55 but she declined the last invitation to attend. She did not want to be a 'difficult patient' but she found the examination to be too uncomfortable. Her husband is 68 years old and has been in a nursing home for the last year following a stroke. He had another stroke 2 months ago and she is worried that the stress of this event has

Obstetrics and Gynaecology: Clinical Cases Uncovered.
By M. Cruickshank and A. Shetty. Published 2009 by Blackwell Publishing. ISBN 978-1-4051-8671-1.

Box 6.1 Tamoxifen

Tamoxifen is a non-steroidal oestrogen antagonist which is used widely as adjuvant treatment for women who have oestrogen receptor positive breast carcinoma. It reduces the risk of recurrence particularly during the first 5 years of treatment, decreases the overall progression of the disease and prevents disease in the contralateral breast. Long-term tamoxifen use is controversial because of its oestrogenic effects on the endometrium. Although it acts as an anti-oestrogen on breast cancer cells, it has a mild oestrogenic effect on the endometrium, bone and cardiovascular system.

Long-term use is associated with proliferative endometrium and a spectrum of benign and malignant changes of the endometrium have been reported including hyperplasia, polyps and carcinoma. The incidence of endometrial carcinoma in the post-menopausal women taking tamoxifen is significantly higher than women not on tamoxifen. Overall, the benefits of tamoxifen against breast cancer recurrence are greater than the risks of developing endometrial cancer.

EB is appropriate as the first line of investigation but you need to remember that a negative result is not conclusive. This will require further investigation by hysteroscopy. TV US appearances can be misleading as tamoxifen can give a sonotranslucent effect on both the endometrial stroma and myometrium. This results in false positive reports in cases of cystic atrophy which appears as thickened cystic endometrium on scan. Histology will confirm multiple cystic spaces lined by atrophic epithelium.

Hysteroscopy is the investigation of choice for women with PMB and a history of tamoxifen usage. It allows direct inspection of the endometrium and full-thickness biopsies using a resectoscope can be taken at the same procedure.

caused her to bleed. She has not been sexually active since.

What would you look for on examination to aid your diagnosis?
Abdominal examination

There are unlikely to be any findings that will aid your diagnosis. Endometrial cancer usually presents with early stage disease which is confined to the uterus. It is rare for endometrial cancer to present at an advanced stage when there may be an omental cake (from tumour infiltration), peritoneal disease, liver enlargement or ascites.

Genital examination

It is important to look for local causes for bleeding including examination of the vulva. It is essential to perform a speculum examination to inspect the vagina and cervix. The finding of a clinical cervical cancer will prompt you to make an urgent referral. A bimanual examination may not be revealing. The uterus is small in postmenopausal women. Uterine enlargement may be incidental (e.g. caused by old calcified fibroids) and the uterus is not usually enlarged with a very early stage endometrial cancer. Less common are ovarian cysts, fibrothecomas, which produce oestrogen which causes endometrial hyperplasia and possible cancer. These ovarian tumours are benign and have the consistency of a fibroid on palpation. They are firm, well defined and mobile. However, it may be difficult to palpate the adnexa in postmenopausal women who find vaginal examinations uncomfortable. Obesity will also make pelvic examination difficult and you may not be able to feel the uterus clearly.

On examination, her vulva is normal and she has mild atrophic changes of her vagina and her cervix. She has some laxity of the vaginal walls but no significant prolapse. She has a small anteverted mobile uterus. You are unable to feel any adnexal masses.

Now review the possible causes of postmenopausal bleeding

• *Endometrial cancer.* You cannot exclude endometrial cancer from the history and examination and you need to consider further investigations.
• *Atrophic vaginitis.* You have found atrophic changes but you still need to exclude other pathology before you can attribute her symptoms to this. This can be treated by topical (intravaginal cream or pessary) oestrogens.
• *Local cervical lesion.* You have excluded local lesions such as a cervical polyp on your examination. Remember that 'ectopy' is related to high oestrogen levels and you should be suspicious of such a finding in a postmenopausal patient.
• *Cervical cancer.* Although she did not attend for her last smear, she has a previous negative screen history and you have not found a clinical cancer. As you have to perform a speculum examination, you should ask her if

you can take a smear to keep her screening up to date (not to diagnose cancer).

• *Iatrogenic.* She has not taken any medication that may cause vaginal bleeding.

• *Chlamydia infection.* You do not need to pursue this as she has not been sexually active in the last year.

• *Stress (as suggested by Mrs Riglinski).* Although some woman may relate bleeding to a stressful event, this does not cause PMB.

What further investigations must you now consider?

Women with PMB can be investigated effectively as outpatients.

Transvaginal ultrasound scanning

Transvaginal ultrasound (TV US) is an accurate method of excluding endometrial cancer. TV US identifies those women who need further investigation by endometrial biopsy (EB) on the basis of the scan findings. Findings that require further investigation by EB:

• Women with an endometrial thickness >4–5 mm (the exact cut-off will depend on local protocols)

• An irregular endometrial outline

• Fluid in the uterine cavity

Fifty percent of postmenopausal women scanned for the investigation of PMB will have a thin regular endometrium and can be reassured at this first visit that no further investigation is required. The negative predictive value is almost 100% in excluding endometrial cancer. This reduces the need for further intervention and allows you to provide reassurance for those women with a normal result.

Report of TV US results for Mrs Riglinski (Fig. 6.1). The uterus contains a regular thickening measuring 8 mm in thickness. This could represent a polyp. Neither ovary can be identified and there are no adnexal masses or free fluid.

What do you do next?

As her endometrial thickness is >4 mm, she requires further investigation. It is often not possible to clearly delineate normal atrophic postmenopausal ovaries. The aim of the scan is to look at the endometrial thickness and outline, although the sonographer may comment on other pelvic structures.

1 *Endometrial biopsy.* There are a number of different devices for obtaining an outpatient EB. If the scan finding represents a polyp, it is unlikely to be removed by EB.

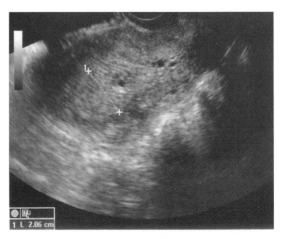

Figure 6.1 Transvaginal ultrasound scan result for Mrs Riglinski.

2 *Hysteroscopy.* Hysteroscopy is often used to investigate PMB as it allows direct inspection of the endometrium. It can detect intrauterine abnormalities and is a sensitive means of identifying polyps and submucous macroscopic findings. It can be used in the outpatient setting using a paracervical block for anaesthetic. Outpatient hysteroscopy is highly acceptable to women. Alternatively, it can be performed under general anaesthetic.

Mrs Riglinski agrees to have an outpatient hysteroscopy with a paracervical block. At hysteroscopy, the cervical canal is normal, the uterine cavity is smooth and regular with a fundal polyp. Both uterine coruna are seen. The polyp is removed using biopsy forceps and sent for histology (Fig. 6.2).

> **KEY POINT**
>
> You need to identify the tubal cornuae to confirm that the hysterocope is in the uterine cavity.

The report from the pathology laboratory confirms a simple endometrial polyp with no evidence of hyperplasia or malignancy.

What further management is required?

Mrs Riglinski does not require any further treatment. Polyp formation after the menopause can be related to tamoxifen or oestrogens. As she is not on HRT this may be related to obesity because of peripheral conversion of androgens (androstenidione) in subcutaneous fat to oestrogens. Polyps may recur but there is no need for follow-

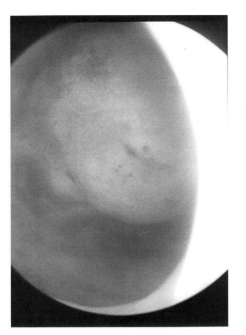

Figure 6.2 Hysteroscopic findings of the endometrial cavity containing a polyp.

up. You should advise Mrs Riglinski to contact her GP if she has further PMB occurring 6 months after her investigations for polyp removal. Remember to warn Mrs Riglinski that it is normal to have some spotting or discharge following the removal of the polyp.

What would have been the management if she was found to have an endometrial cancer?

Women with endometrial cancer confined to the uterus are usually curable by surgery and most women present with early stage disease. The treatment of choice is total abdominal hysterectomy and bilateral salpingo-oopherectomy (TAH/BSO) with peritoneal washings taken on opening the abdominal cavity for staging cytology.

When there is deep myometrial invasion or grade 3 disease, the prognosis with standard surgery alone is poorer because of the risk of spread to pelvic lymph nodes and recurrence. Endometrial cancer is radiosensitive and cure can still be achieved in early stage disease. Radiotherapy may also be given following surgery for women considered at increased risk of recurrent disease. Adjuvant radiotherapy is given to treat the pelvis by external beam with a caesium insertion to the vaginal vault and/or chemotherapy.

Women with endometrial cancer are often elderly with other medical problems and preoperative assessment for fitness for an anaesthetic and surgery is essential.

CASE REVIEW

Postmenopausal bleeding is defined as bleeding more than 12 months since a woman's last normal period. However, women who continue to menstruate after the age of 55 years, who have unscheduled bleeds on cyclical HRT or continue to bleed more than 6 months after starting continuous combined HRT also need to be investigated.

Transvaginal ultrasound scan should be the first line investigation as it allows good views of the pelvis and the endometrium. Transabdominal scanning may be used for the few women who cannot tolerate the intravaginal probe. Women with an endometrium measuring 5 mm or greater are at increased risk of endometrial cancer and require an endometrial biopsy. This can be performed at the same visit using an endometrial sampler. However, if the specimen is inadequate for histology, cancer has not been excluded and a hysteroscopy and biopsy are required to obtain an adequate biopsy or confirm

the absence of endometrial pathology. Hysteroscopy should also be performed if an endometrial polyp is suspected on TV US.

Women with a history of taking tamoxifen, especially for longer than 5 years, are at increased risk of endometrial polyps, cancer and sarcoma. However, the effects on the endometrium and myometrium mean that TV US is not reliable and a hysteroscopy and full-thickness biopsy are essential to exclude cancer. Women who are asymptomatic on tamoxifen do not need to be investigated or screened for endometrial cancer.

Once endometrial cancer has been excluded, any local causes can be treated. Often reassurance is all that is required. Following investigation, women should be re-referred for further investigation if they continue to experience PMB after 6 months.

KEY POINTS

- Women with PMB need to be investigated to exclude endometrial cancer
- About 8–10% of women with PMB will have endometrial cancer
- A further 1–2% will have a malignancy at another site, e.g. cervix, vulva, bladder or anus
- Visual inspection of the cervix is essential to identify cervical cancer
- TV US is an accurate method of excluding endometrial cancer and provides rapid reassurance to women with a thin and regular endometrium

- Women with a endometrial thickness >5 mm or an irregular contour require further investigation by endometrial biopsy +/– hysteroscopy
- Women with unscheduled bleeds on HRT need to be investigated
- Women on continuous combined HRT may initially have irregular bleeding but need to be investigated if this continues beyond 6 months
- The benefits of tamoxifen in breast cancer treatment outweigh the risks but any abnormal vaginal bleeding while on tamoxifen requires full investigation

---

Further reading

Investigation of Post Menopausal Bleeding. SIGN Guideline Publication 61.ISBN 1899893 13 X. September 2002.

A couple who cannot conceive

A 25-year-old hairdresser, Mina Blackburn, presented with her 28-year-old husband, Chris, an offshore engineer, because of their inability to conceive over the last 12 months. She stopped depo-medroxyprogesterone acetate injections (DMPA) a year ago. She has never been pregnant before. Her menstrual cycle is irregular. When her husband is home she frequently uses ovulation kits. She is very anxious and feels that there is something wrong with her. Her distress is increased by the fact that her younger sister had a 20-week scan showing a twin pregnancy last week.

What information should you elicit from the history?

History from the female partner
- Menstrual history:
  - detail of length and regularity of her cycle
  - how was her cycle prior to using DMPA?
  - how long she has been on DMPA?
  - any history of dysmenorrhoea?
- Has she ever tried for pregnancy in any previous relationship?
- History of any alterations in weight
- Past history of pelvic inflammatory diseases, *Chlamydia* or any other sexually transmitted infection
- Any significant past medical or surgical history or drug allergies
- Timing and result of most recent cervical smear test

History from male partner
- Has he fathered any pregnancies before?
- How frequently he works offshore? Does he work near heat?

- Any surgery (specifically testicular torsion, orchipexy, appendectomy)
- Any history of mumps

History from both partners
- Intercourse: frequency, dysparunia, problems with ejaculation
- History of smoking and alcohol use

Mina had menarche at the age of 13 years, since then she had a regular cycle. She used the combined oral contraceptive for contraception from the age of 16 years for 5 years but changed to DMPA as she did not have to remember to take it. She met her present partner at the age of 22 years and the couple decided to try for pregnancy so Mina did not continue with DMPA. She admits that she has gained 2 stones (12.7 kg) in weight over last 2 years and her body mass index (BMI) is 33 in the clinic today. Since coming off DMPA her periods have not been regular.

Chris has not fathered any children. He denies a history of mumps or any genital surgery. He is fit and healthy. He works offshore with a rota of 4 weeks off and 4 weeks on. He does not work near heat, radiation or chemicals. The last year has been particularly stressful for the couple as Chris had to be away from home for much of his time onshore as his mother has been very ill. With a change in his job plan, he will be office-based onshore from next month.

The couple deny any problems with sexual intercourse. They are both non-smokers and have the occasional glass of wine.

What are the issues to consider in this case?

Actual length of time trying for pregnancy
As Chris is away more than half of the time, the duration of unprotected sex does not amount to 12 months. Subfertility is defined as inability to conceive after 1 year of regular unprotected intercourse.

Obstetrics and Gynaecology: Clinical Cases Uncovered.
By M. Cruickshank and A. Shetty. Published 2009 by Blackwell Publishing. ISBN 978-1-4051-8671-1.

Mina's weight gain

Increased BMI is associated with anovulation or ovulatory dysfunction.

Use of DMPA

Return to fertility is not immediate after coming off DMPA. It can take up to 6–9 months after the last injection.

What initial advice would you give to the couple?
Reassurance

About 84% of couples in the general population will conceive within 1 year if they do not use contraception and have regular sexual intercourse. Of those who do not conceive in the first year, about half will do so in the second year.

With the actual length (less than 1 year) of trying for conception this couple is still within the favourable time zone. Chris's job change to onshore gives the couple a relatively high chance of spontaneous conception.

Advice on weight loss

Mina's irregular periods suggest infrequent ovulation. The fact that Mina gained 2 stones in weight in recent years can explain ovulatory dysfunction and irregular cycles. She should be strongly advised to lose weight. Even losing 5–10% of body weight can regulate periods, enhance the chances of spontaneous pregnancy and decreases the risk of miscarriage. In addition, it improves general well-being. Participating in a group programme involving dietary advice and exercises will improve weight loss compared to advice alone.

Intercourse

Sexual intercourse every 2–3 days optimizes the chance of pregnancy. Timing intercourse to coincide with ovulation causes stress and is not recommended. Ovulation kits are based on luteinizing hormone (LH) peak around ovulation.

Folic acid

As Mina is trying to become pregnant she should be advised to take folic acid (0.4 mg/day) to reduce the risk of neural tube defects.

What further investigations should you consider?
Male partner
Semen analysis

This should be the first test in infertility investigations as up to 40% of men can have suboptimal semen parameters (as per World Health Organization reference range; Table 7.1).

Female partner
Immunity to rubella

Rubella screening is recommended so that those who are susceptible can be offered vaccination. Women should be advised not to become pregnant for at least 1 month following vaccination and a repeat serum sample should be taken to confirm immunity.

Basal hormonal profile

As her cycle is irregular, basal follicle stimulating hormone (FSH), LH, prolactin (PRL), thyroid function test (TFT) and serum testosterone tests should be peformed. Timing of these tests need to be specified as

Table 7.1 WHO reference values for semen analysis 2000.

Criteria	Reference values
Volume	2.0 mL or more
Liquefaction time	Within 60 minutes
pH	7.2 or more
Sperm concentration	20 million spermatozoa per millilitre or more
Total sperm number	40 million spermatozoa per ejaculate or more
Motility	50% or more motile (grade a + b) or >25% grade a within 60 minutes of ejaculation (motility is graded as a–d. Grade a, rapid progressive motility; grade b, slow progressive motility; grade c, non-progressive motility; grade d, immotile)
Morphology	15%
While blood cells	Less than 1 million per millilitre

basal, that is day 1–5 of her menstrual cycle (day 1 is the day of starting her period).

> **KEY POINT**
>
> Assessment of ovulation by mid-luteal progesterone is not recommended as her cycle is irregular and the mid-luteal phase cannot be determined.

Transvaginal ultrasound

Transvaginal scan of the female partner is recommended to rule out polycystic ovaries and to have baseline assessment of her uterus.

Urinary *Chlamydia* test

A urine *Chlamydia* test is used to screen for infection. *Chlamydia* is a common cause of infertility from tubal blockage. *Chlamydia trachomatis* is present in 10% of the sexually active population aged 19 years or less. It is a major cause of pelvic inflammatory disease, leading to chronic abdominal pain, ectopic pregnancy and tubal factor infertility. Asymptomatic *Chlamydia* infection may go unrecognized and untreated. Although the prevalence of *Chlamydia* among subfertile women in the UK is only 1.9%, uterine instrumentation carried out routinely as part of infertility investigation may reactivate or introduce upper tract dissemination of an endocervical *Chlamydia* infection, resulting in iatrogenic pelvic inflammatory disease. DNA techniques such as polymerase chain reaction and ligase chain reaction for analysis of cervical and urine specimens are highly sensitive and specific for diagnosing *Chlamydia* infection.

> **KEY POINT**
>
> All patients who may require cervical instrumentation should be screened for *Chlamydia* so that if present, the infection is not exacerbated.

The couple return after 4 months. Chris works onshore all the time. Mina has managed to lose 3 kg in weight. Her FSH, LH, PRL, TFT and testosterone are all within normal limits. A pelvic ultrasound at the last visit

showed evidence of polycystic ovaries. Her urine Chlamydia test is negative. Her menstrual cycle is more regular at κ = 4–5/30–37 days. The result of Chris's semen analysis is as follows:

Volume	*2.0 mL*
Liquefaction time	*45 minutes*
pH	*7.3*
Sperm concentration	*18 million/mL*
Total sperm number	*36 million*

Sperm motility:

grade a	*10%*
grade b	*15%*
grade c	*35%*
grade d	*40%*
White blood cell	*none*
Morphology	*7%*

Chris is completely devastated to be told that his semen parameters are suboptimal causing infertility.

What advice will you give the couple at this visit?

You should try to reassure the couple. The test for semen analysis is a very poor predictor of fertility. It is a sensitive test but the specificity is very low. An abnormal test does not always mean true abnormality. Check that he followed the instructions for semen analysis correctly:

- He did not miss the receptacle for collecting the specimen
- The couple abstained from intercourse for at least 72 hours
- Any history of recent viral illness
- The sample reached laboratory in time
- The sample was not exposed to heat or cold before reaching the laboratory
- He is not on any medication

What should you do now?

A repeat sample should be requested at least 3 weeks after the last sample. A single test will falsely identify about 10% of men as abnormal, but repeating the test reduces this to 2%. However, if the first semen analysis is normal then there is no need to repeat it.

Now review the situation for this couple

Mina has a regular cycle now and you need to check that she is ovulating. Ovulation is checked by mid-luteal progesterone (traditionally called day 21 progesterone). As the length of the secretary phase is constant to 14 days, mid-luteal progesterone has to be timed according to the luteal phase and length of the cycle. The cycle length minus 7 is the day mid-luteal progesterone should be checked to detect ovulation. In this case you can start tracking her progesterone from day 23 and can repeat it in 7 days' time (as Mina's cycle length = 30–37 days; day 23 for 30-day cycle and day 30 for 37-day cycle). Values range 16–28 nmol/L as the lowest limit is suggestive of ovulation. In the meantime, encourage the couple to keep trying for a pregnancy.

Mid-luteal progesterone shows the highest value of 10 nmol/L. The repeat semen analysis is as follows:

Volume	*3.0 mL*
Liquefaction time	*45 minutes*
pH	*7.3*
Sperm concentration	*25 million/mL*
Total sperm number	*75 million*
Sperm motility:	
grade a	*25%*
grade b	*5%*
grade c	*30%*
grade d	*40%*
White blood cell	*none*
Morphology	*15%*

You see the couple to discuss these results. What information can you give them based on the results of their investigations?

• Repeat investigations have revealed normal semen parameters
• Serum progesterone level indicates anovulation
• The diagnosis of polycystic ovarian syndrome is made as per the Rotterdam criteria (international consensus). This criterion requires the presence of two out of three of the following criteria:
  ○ oligomenorrhoea or anovulation
  ○ clinical and biochemical hyperandrogenism
  ○ polycystic ovaries on ultrasound (at least 12 follicles measuring 2–9 mm in diameter and or an ovarian volume in excess of 10 cm³)

What are the clinical implications for this couple?

In this case the diagnosis is oligovulation or anovulation as well as ultrasound features of polycystic ovaries.

Treatment consists of:
• Ovulation induction when the patient wishes to conceive
• Encourage her to continue to lose weight
• Ovulation induction because a diagnosis of anovulation has been made (Box 7.1)

Box 7.1 Ovulation induction

• Clomiphene citrate is the first line of drug for ovulation induction in women with anovulation
• It is an anti-oestrogen and induces gonadotrophin release by occupying the oestrogen receptors in the hypothalamus, thereby interfering with the normal feedback mechanism. Increased gonadotrophins stimulate the ovaries to produce more follicles
• It is associated with the adverse effects of hot flushes, ovarian hyperstimulation, abdominal discomfort and multiple pregnancies
• Clomiphene is started at a dose of 50 mg/day for 5 days
• You need to monitor at least the first cycle by pelvic ultrasound scan to check how many follicles are developing
• If three or more follicles develop, you advise the patient to use contraception in order to avoid a multiple pregnancy
• Evidence of ovulation is checked by measuring mid-luteal progesterone or tracking follicles on ultrasound
• The dosage is increased in the subsequent cycle if ovulation is not documented. Approximately 70–80% of anovulatory women ovulate on clomiphene at the dose of 100–150 mg; however, only 30–40% become pregnant
• If pregnancy is not achieved after three ovulatory cycles on clomiphene, a check for tubal patency is now indicated

---

KEY POINT

You do not need to check for tubal patency prior to ovulation induction. There is nothing in the history suggestive of tubal damage or pelvic inflammatory disease, and her *Chlamydia* test was negative.

After 4 months Mina attends your clinic for review. She had three cycles of clomiphene at 100mg, all of which have been documented as ovulatary. However, she did not become pregnant.

What would you do next?
You need to check the patency of her fallopian tubes using one of the following methods.

Hysterosalpingography
This is an outpatient-based investigation in which a radio-opaque dye is passed through the cervix and an X-ray of the pelvis is taken to look for dye spill from the fimbrial end of the tube. In addition, it supplies imaging information about uterine abnormality as the cavity is visualized.

Diagnostic laparoscopy and dye test
This is the gold standard for diagnosis of tubal occlusion. It gives information on pelvic or tubal adhesions, the presence of endometriosis and fibroids as well as determining tubal patency. However, laparoscopy involves general anaesthesia, and is associated with a small risk of bowel injury.

Hysterosalpingocontrast sonography
This is an outpatient-based procedure where contrast agent is passed through the cervix and the tubes are visualized on ultrasound.

The couple decide to go ahead with a laparoscopy and dye test. Mina is found to have a normal pelvis and both fallopian tubes are patent. Afterwards, a plan is agreed to continue with clomiphene citrate for further two cycles. Following the second cycle, Mina misses her period and a urinary pregnancy test is positive. She has a 8-week scan showing an intrauterine ongoing pregnancy (singleton).

CASE REVIEW

When most couples reach the fertility clinic they are very distressed and the situation is compounded by the fact that everyone around them seems to become pregnant without any problems. They need an empathetic approach rather than just a barrage of investigations. Stress is known to reduce fertility; lifestyle modification including weight reduction and promoting a healthy lifestyle should be part of the initial approach while investigating for other causes.

As all the investigations, especially semen analysis, are very poor predictors of fertility, the couple need to be counselled that numbers not matching with reference range does not mean sterility. There may be other factors responsible. However, it is reassuring if all the investigations are normal (mid-luteal progesterone documenting ovulation, normal semen analysis and patent fallopian tubes) but it can be frustrating if there is no cause to explain their subfertility.

Approximately 20% of the couples attending infertility clinics fall into this category. Treatments for unexplained infertility are largely empirical and include superovulation and intrauterine insemination (stimulating ovaries with gonadotrophins and timing semen insemination once the follicle is mature). Ovulatory dysfunction is largely treated by medical means (clomiphene citrate and/or gonadotrophins).

If there is suspicion of tubal blockage (such as a history of *Chlamydia*, or other sexually transmitted diseases), patency of the tubes should be checked before commencing on ovulation-inducing drugs. If tubes are blocked, *in vitro* fertilization (IVF) is a more cost effective treatment than tubal surgery.

KEY POINTS

- Lifestyle modifications should be first line of approach
- Reassurance and support are important aspects of care
- Aim of the investigations is to identify the cause of infertility (tubal, anovulatory, male factor or unexplained)
- Rubella immunity must be checked for all women trying to conceive
- Mid-luteal progesterone may not always be on day 21. It depends on the length of the menstrual cycle
- Clomiphene citrate is first line of treatment for ovulatory dysfunction
- IVF is a cost effective option for tubal blockage
- Treatments for unexplained infertility are largely empirical
- There are no proven medical treatments for sperm disorders

Case 8 | A 16-year-old seeking emergency contraception: contraceptive choices through reproductive life

Louise is 16 years old and has dropped into her local sexual health clinic to pick up condoms. She has been seeing Tom for 5 weeks and two nights ago they had unprotected sex. Louise knows that this puts her at risk of pregnancy and is frightened. She is studying for her A-levels and plans to go to university. Pregnancy would be a disaster for her.

What could reduce Louise's risk of pregnancy?

She could take emergency contraception (EC). There are two options: oral (levonorgestrel (1500 μg)) or the intra-uterine device (IUD).

Louise has heard something about the 'morning after pill' but she was not sure where to get it and she thinks it is too late to use this.

The 'morning after pill' is a misnomer for EC which can be taken up to 72 hours (3 days) after unprotected sex and in some cases up to 120 hours (5 days) after ovulation.

What other information do you need to know in order to give EC safely?

• *The date of her last menstrual period (LMP).* Her risk of pregnancy depends on what day in her cycle she had unprotected sexual intercourse:
  ○ days 8–17 = 20–30% risk of pregnancy
  ○ days 1–7 and >17 = 2–3% risk of pregnancy
• The date and time of any episodes of unprotected sexual intercourse since her LMP and how many hours have elapsed. You need to establish if it is over 72 hours.
• *Medical and drug history.* Taking a liver enzyme inducer drug means the dose of levonorgestrel needs to

be doubled (Box 8.1). An IUD would be better in this situation.
• *Prior use of emergency contraception.* You need to ask if she had vomiting or an allergic reaction.

Louise has never used EC before. She has no relevant past medical history and is not on any drugs. She had unprotected sexual intercourse 54 hours ago on day 11 of a regular 28-day cycle. The sex was consensual. She and Tom have been using condoms but forgot on that occasion. She had no other unprotected episodes since her period.

What important points need to be raised about each method before Louise can make a choice?
Oral EC: 1500 μg levonorgestrel

The efficacy depends on the time taken:
• Within 24 hours of unprotected sexual intercourse = 95% reduction in expected pregnancies
• Within 25–48 hours of unprotected sexual intercourse = 85% reduction in expected pregnancies
• Within 49–72 hours of unprotected sexual intercourse = 58% reduction in expected pregnancies

Nausea is common (14%) and 1% of women taking EC vomit. If she vomits within 2 hours, she needs a further dose together with an antiemetic. If her next

---

> **Box 8.1 Liver enzyme inducing drugs**
>
> Rifampicin
> Rifabutin
> St John's wort
> Griseofulvin
> Anticonvulsants (phenytoin, carbamazepine, barbiturates, primidone, topiramate, oxcarbazepine)
> Tacrolimus
> Certain antiretroviral (HIV) drugs

Obstetrics and Gynaecology: Clinical Cases Uncovered.
By M. Cruickshank and A. Shetty. Published 2009 by Blackwell Publishing. ISBN 978-1-4051-8671-1.

period is lighter or absent, she needs to do a urine pregnancy test. You need to advise her to abstain from sex until her next period.

Copper IUD

• >99% reduction in expected pregnancies
• Immediate contraception
• She needs to return after her next period for removal or thread check if she plans to continue to use it
• IUD can be given up to 5 days after unprotected sexual intercourse or 120 hours after expected ovulation (day 19 in Louise's case)

> **KEY POINT**
>
> The intrauterine system (IUS) cannot be used for EC.

Louise does not like the idea of an IUD and opts for oral EC.

What else would you like to discuss with her?

• Her intended contraception use.
• Her risk of sexually transmitted infection (STI). Consider *Chlamydia* screening +/− antibiotic prophylaxis (1 g azithromycin) if at risk of STI.

What contraceptive methods could Louise use?

From the history so far, Louise is suitable for all methods. You could show her a leaflet outlining all her choices.

What specific information would you like to know to aid her decision?

1 *Contraindications to taking oestrogen*:
  ○ Multiple risk factors for arterial cardiovascular disease (CVD) (e.g. smoking, diabetes, hypertension, ischaemic heart disease, stroke, complicated heart disease)
  ○ Personal or close family history of venous thromboembolism (VTE)
  ○ Migraine with aura
  ○ Breast cancer or carrier of *BRCA* gene mutation
  ○ Gall bladder and liver disease/tumours
  ○ BMI => 35
  ○ A sustained systolic blood pressure (BP) of >140 or diastolic of >90 mmHg

2 *Her menstrual history.* Certain methods make periods lighter, more regular, less painful and can help premenstrual symptoms.
3 *Lifestyle.* Some long-acting reversible contraceptive (LARC) methods would particularly suit those working shifts or crossing time zones.
4 *Which methods would she not consider?*
  ○ Combined oral contraception (COC) and progesterone only pill (POP) may not be suitable if she finds swallowing tablets difficult
  ○ Depo-medroxyprogesterone acetate (DMPA) and progesterone only implant (POI) if needle-phobic as they require a needle insertion
  ○ The IUD, IUS and diaphragm/cap may be difficult to fit if she has difficulty with vaginal examinations

What examinations do you need to do?

• Height and weight for BMI
• Blood pressure

Louise has no relevant medical, family or drug history, has a BMI of 28 and a BP of 120/78 mmHg.

What are her options?

• DMPA
• IUD
• IUS
• COC/patch
• POP or POI
• Barrier methods

What options would not be advisable?

Male or female sterilization is not suitable as these are irreversible.

What key counselling points would you include to help Louise decide the best method for her?

See Table 8.1.

How is the implant inserted?

This is inserted with local anaesthetic under the skin in the medial aspect of the upper part of the non-dominant arm. It should be easily palpable.

Table 8.1 Advantages and disadvantages of methods of long-acting reversible contraception.

	Advantages	Disadvantages	
DMPA	Very effective	Injection	UK MEC recommends other methods if a patient is <18 or >45 years
	Inhibits ovulation	Irregular bleeding common first few months	
	Administered every 12 weeks	Expect weight gain of 2–3 kg/year	Limited evidence shows a decrease in BMD during use, but gained back on discontinuation
	Periods usually absent after third injection	Progestogenic side-effects common (acne, bloating, breast tenderness and mood change)	
	May improve dysmenorrhoea and protect against uterine cancer and PID		Peak bone mass is achieved during the teen years
	Contraceptive effect lasts 14 weeks	Reduced BMD while using	
		Periods and fertility may take a number of months to return to normal	
		Does not protect against STIs	
POI	Lasts for 3 years	Bleeding pattern is unpredictable: 20% amenorrhoea, 40% unusual pattern, 40% irregular bleeding	Etonogestrel flexible rod measuring 4 cm × 2 mm
	Rapid return of fertility on removal		
	Very effective	Progestogenic side-effects common	
	Inhibits ovulation	Does not protect against STIs	
	Some protection against PID and uterine cancer	Rarely, removal difficult	

BMD, bone mineral density; DMPA, depo-medroxyprogesterone acetate; PID, pelvic inflammatory disease; POI, progesterone only implant; STI, sexually transmitted infection; UK MEC, Medical Eligibility Criteria.

Louise has a friend who had a POI, but she had it removed as she bled all the time.

What would you advise Louise?

Bleeding problems with progesterone only methods (DMPA, POI, POP and IUS) are very common and can lead to discontinuation and risk of pregnancy. Counselling must give realistic expectations. Unpredictable bleeding (heavy, spotting or prolonged) may occur but usually improves over 6 months. You can add the COC for cycle control or a non-steroidal anti-inflammatory drug such as mefenamic acid.

Louise does not like needles and wants to know about pills.

What are the differences between combined oral contraception and progestogen only pills?

See Table 8.2.

Many of Louise's friends take the COC. Which would you consider starting her on?

- Microgynon 30
- Loestrin

These contain levonorgestrel or norethisterone. While the COC has an increased risk of VTE, the absolute risk is very small. When prescribing for the first time, however, always try to prescribe the drug with the lowest risk (Box 8.2).

Table 8.2 Comparison of combined oral contraceptive (COC) and progesterone only pill (POP).

	COC	POP
What is in it?	Ethinyl oestradiol and a progestogen	Progestogen only
Advantages	Regular, lighter periods	No oestrogen
	Reduced period pain	No serious side-effects
	Inhibits ovulation	Inhibits ovulation (Cerazette)
	Protects against ovarian and uterine cancer	
	Avoid periods by running packs together (outside product licence)	
Disadvantages	Minor side-effects: nausea, headache (if these are focal COC would be contraindicated), breakthrough bleeding, discharge and mood changes	Minor side-effects: progestogenic and unpredictable bleeding
	Serious side-effects rare but include: VTE, MI, ischaemic strike, cervical cancer and possibly breast cancer	May be less effective if >70 kg – recommend two tablets per day (one tablet if Cerazette)
		Tight dosage timing (not Cerazette)
		The newest POP Cerazette has advantages over traditional POPs in that, like the COC, it has a 12-hour dosage widow (compared to 3 hours) and inhibits ovulation
How to take	1 tablet for 21 days and then a 7-day break	1 tablet every day

MI, myocardial infarction; VTE, venous thromboembolism.

Box 8.2 Risk of venous thromboembolism

Non-combined oral contraception (COC) users	5 per 100,000 woman years
Levonorgestrel or norethisterone containing COC	15 per 100,000 woman years
Desogestrel or gestodene containing COC	25 per 100,000 woman years
Pregnancy	60 per 100,000 woman years

Louise's older sister uses the patch. What advantages does it have over COC?

Compliance is easier as one patch is applied once a week rather than taking one pill per day. Absorption is not affected by vomiting, diarrhoea or antibiotics. Some women can develop a skin reaction to the adhesive.

At this stage you ask Louise if she would like to discuss non-hormonal methods.

Are these methods really an option for Louise?

Male condoms are readily available and have an important role in safe sex. On their own, however, they have a high failure rates in teenagers when fertility is at its peak. Female condoms are expensive, noisy and need to be fitted prior to sex. This makes them unpopular with teenagers.

Diaphragms, caps and natural family planning (NFP) require considerable motivation and are rarely used by this age group.

Young age and no previous delivery do not preclude use of the IUS or IUD but they are not popular methods in this age group. Fitting often requires a local anaesthetic. STI screening is usually required before insertion, and safe sex advised.

Louise agrees on the COC and you also give her free condoms and advice on safer sex.

Would you offer her anything else?

A *Chlamydia* test. Her age confers a 10% risk of *Chlamydia* infection. The majority of *Chlamydia* infections are asymptomatic and unrecognized infections can cause PID which can lead to ectopic pregnancy, tubal factor infertility and pelvic pain.

Nine years later, Louise is 25 and has been on DMPA for 2 years. She is considering a break from hormonal contraception. She and her partner Bob have been together for 2 years. She is nulliparous.

> **KEY POINT**
>
> The Medicines and Healthcare Products Regulatory Agency recommends that females should be reviewed after 2 years of DMPA in order to re-evaluate the risks and benefits of continuing use in view of its effect on bone mineral density (BMD).

What are her non-hormonal contraceptive options?

- IUD
- Male and female condoms
- Diaphragm/cap with spermicide
- NFP

What further information do you need to assess suitability?
IUD

You need to ask if she has had any other partners in the past year to assess her risk of STIs. Contraindications include pregnancy, copper allergy, unexplained vaginal bleeding and uterine abnormalities.

Diaphragm/cap

Does she have a history of urinary tract infections (UTIs)? Is she is comfortable touching her own genitals to fit the cap?

Natural family planning

Is her mentrual cycle regular? Can she commit to daily monitoring and charting? Is she aware of the failure rate?

Louise is interested in the IUD or diaphragm.

What main counselling points would you raise? She and Bob are planning to travel for 6 months. Does this affect your counselling?
IUD

- *Advantages:*
  - highly effective
  - immediate action
  - lasts for up to 10 years
  - rapid return of fertility on removal
  - no hormones
  - no drug interactions
- *Disadvantages:*
  - during insertion the IUD can, rarely, perforate and enter the abdominal cavity
  - there is a small chance of infection during the first 20 days following insertion
  - the IUD can expel in 5% of cases, most commonly in the first 3 months of use
  - if the device fails, there is a 20% chance the pregnancy will be ectopic
  - periods can become heavier, longer and more painful. Intermenstrual bleeding is also common
- *Follow-up:*
  - check at 3–6 weeks to view threads
  - women are advised to check threads after each period or at regular intervals
- *Removal:*
  - anytime, by pulling gently at threads. Ask patients to abstain from sex or use condoms for a week before to avoid possible pregnancy.

For women who travel the IUD is 'forgettable' and cannot get lost. There is no oestrogen so there is no increased risk of a VTE.

> **KEY POINT**
>
> An IUD is suitable for nulliparous women. Prior to insertion, consider STI swabs in women under 25 years or those with a new partner in last 3 months or more than one partner in the past year.

Diaphragm

- *Advantages:*
  - over 90% efficacy if used correctly
  - hormone free
  - no drug interactions
  - some protection against STIs
- *Disadvantages:*
  - needs to be put in before sex
  - spermicide can be messy
  - UTIs can be a problem with diaphragms
  - correct insertion needs to be taught
  - latex diaphragms and caps can be damaged by oil-based products
- *How is it fitted:*
  - a trained fitter performs a vaginal examination and chooses from a range of diaphragms
  - the fitter tries a suitable size and model and then gets the patient to insert it
  - the patient returns 1–2 weeks later with it inserted to check the fit

For women who travel the diaphragm offers some protection against STIs but condoms would also be recommended. There is no oestrogen so there is no increased risk of a VTE. Spermicide might prove difficult to access in remote areas.

Louise is now 35 years old and has used the IUD on and off for 15 years. She has three children and feels that her family is complete. Her youngest is 3 months

old and she is exclusively breastfeeding with no periods. Her relationship with Bob is strained but they are still together. She had a ruptured appendix in Thailand when she was travelling which required an open appendicectomy and prolonged recovery. Her periods were getting heavier and more painful. She smokes 10 cigarettes per day and is taking St John's wort for postnatal depression.

Does she need contraception at the moment?

No. Her baby is less than 6 months old, she is exclusively breastfeeding and amenorrhoeic. Lactational amenorrhoea produces 98% natural contraceptive cover. She must be advised that this effectiveness reduces when weaning starts and the amount of breast milk consumed reduces.

From her history, what are the pros and cons for her contraceptive options?

See Table 8.3.

> **KEY POINT**
>
> Vasectomy protocols vary between units, but from around 8 weeks after a vasectomy, a semen kit is mailed out and men are asked to provide a sample of ejaculation to be examined for sperm. Two negative samples are usually requested before the operation is deemed effective and contraception can be stopped.

PART 2: CASES

Table 8.3 Advantages and disadvantages of various types of contraception.

Type	Advantages	Disadvantages
DMPA	High efficacy	Review after 2 years
	Amenorrhoea	Weight gain
	No drug interactions	Unpredictable bleeding
	Suitable while breastfeeding	Progestogenic side-effects
	Suitable for smokers	
	Reversible	
POI	High efficacy	Reduced efficacy with LEIs such as St John's wort
	Lasts 3 years	Unpredictable bleeding
	Suitable for smokers	Progestogenic side-effects
	Suitable while breastfeeding	

Continued on p. 68

Table 8.3 *Continued*

Type	Advantages	Disadvantages
IUS (progestogen-coated IUD)	High efficacy	Unpredictable bleeding common for first 3–6 months
	Lasts 5 years	Progestogenic side-effects
	95% decrease in menses by 3 months	
	65% amenorrhoeic at 1 year	
	Suitable for smokers and breastfeeding	
	No drug interactions	
	Reversible	
IUD	High efficacy	May make periods heavier or more painful but you can consider adding tranexamic acid or NSAID to reduce pain and bleeding
	Suitable for smokers and breastfeeding	
	No drug interactions	
	Reversible	
Female sterilization	Suitable for smokers and breastfeeding	Failure rate 1/200; >DMPA, POI and IUS
	No drug interactions	Usually performed laparoscopically, so risk of vessel and organ damage higher as she has a midline scar
	Periods might improve with removal of IUD	Risk of general anaesthetic
		Postoperative recovery
		Small increased risk of ectopic pregnancy
		Reversal often not funded by the NHS
Male sterilization	Usually performed under local anaesthetic	Takes at least 2 months before effective
	1/2000 failure rate once azoospermia confirmed	Bruising, swelling and pain in scrotum is common
	No effect on erectile function, testicular or prostatic cancer, or CVD	Reversal often not funded by the NHS
COC/patch		Unsuitable for smokers ≥35 years because of increased CVD risk
		Affected adversely by liver enzyme inducers such as St John's wort
		Unsuitable while breastfeeding as may affect breast milk volume
POP	Suitable for smokers and while breastfeeding	Affected by liver enzyme inducers such as St John's wort
		Progestogenic side-effects
		Unpredictable bleeding common
Male and female condoms	See previous section	
	Consider advance provision of EC	

Table 8.3 *Continued*

Type	Advantages	Disadvantages
Diaphragm/cap	See previous section	
	Consider advance provision of EC	
Natural family planning	Up to 98% effective if used according to teaching and instructions	Efficacy user dependent
		Takes up to 6 months to learn
	More effective when taught by a specific NFP teacher	Daily recording
	Examples include cervical secretions, basal temperature, cervical changes (position and consistency)	Events that affect the menstrual cycle (illness, stress, breastfeeding) may make fertility indications more difficult to interpret
	Can help to plan or avoid pregnancy	Fertility motion devices can be purchased from pharmacies or over the Internet but can be expensive
	Hormone free	
	No drug interactions	
	Acceptable to all faiths and cultures	

COC, combined oral contraception; CVD, cardiovascular disease; DMPA, depo-medroxyprogesterone acetate; EC, emergency contraception; IUD, intrauterine device; IUS, intrauterine system; LEI, liver enzyme inducer; NFP, natural family planning; NSAID, non-steroidal anti-inflammatory drug; POI, progesterone only implant; POP, progesterone only pill.

Table 8.4 Contraceptive options for the perimenopausal woman.

DMPA	Amenorrhoea and decreased BMD prior to loss of BMD in the menopause
POI	Unpredictable bleeding may be difficult to differentiate from organic pathology, e.g. endometrial polyps, DUB or endometrial cancer
IUS	Unpredictable bleeding (as POI)
	May help heavy painful periods
	Can be used as the progesterone component of HRT (licensed for 4 years' use)
	If fitted at 45 years old, can be retained for 7 years
IUD	If inserted from 40 years, can remain until the menopause
	May contribute to DUB that needs investigation for alternative pathology
Female sterilization	Midline scar increases risks of surgery at a time when fertility is falling
COC/patch	Unsuitable as she has continued to smoke
	Compared with non-users, COC carries an increased risk of ischemic stroke, MI and VTE, which is magnified considerably by smoking
	Any increased risk of breast cancer is likely to be small

Continued on p. 70

Table 8.4 *Continued*

DMPA	Amenorrhoea and decreased BMD prior to loss of BMD in the menopause
POP	Good efficacy in this age group with reduced fertility
	Safe, so often continued until 55 years
	Unpredictable bleeding may need investigation to rule out pathology
Male condoms	Used effectively in this age group and low fertility improves effectiveness
	Older men have increasing rates of erectile dysfunction and condoms can exacerbate this
Diaphragm	Prolapse may make fitting and use more difficult
	Fluctuating levels of oestrogen may predispose to urethritis and vaginal discomfort

BMD, bone mineral density; COC, combined oral contraceptive; DMPA, depo-medroxypregesterone acetate; DUB, dysfunctional uterine bleeding; HRT, hormone replacement therapy; IUD, intrauterine device; IUS, intrauterine system; MI, myocardial infarction; POI, progesterone only implant; POP, progesterone only pill; VTE, venous thromboembolism.

Louise decided to use DMPA. She is now aged 45 years old and has been amenorrhoeic for a number of years. She and Bob split up 4 years ago. She still smokes and was diagnosed with coeliac disease 2 months ago. She has started experiencing some hot flushes and night sweats. Although she has an occasional partner, Jim, she wants to know when she can stop contraception as she is sure she is 'going through the change'.

What advice would you give her?

The average age for the menopause in the UK is 51 years. As there is a risk of unpredictable ovulation in the peri-menopause, contraception is recommended for 2 years if the menopause is diagnosed before 50 years or for 1 year if a woman is over 50 years. A third option is to continue contraception until 55 years, when 96% of women will be menopausal and infertile.

Her DMPA-induced amenorrhoea, smoking and coeliac disease put her at risk of osteoporosis. She should stop DMPA and should be considered for a bone scan to measure baseline BMD.

What issues in the perimenopause may preclude or recommend a contraceptive option?

See Table 8.4.

CASE REVIEW

Louise presents with contraceptive needs at different ages and different life stages. There are only a finite number of methods available and each will have advantages and disadvantages depending on each individual's circumstances.

Those aged under 20 years have high fertility and are at increased risk of STIs. Condoms are excellent at preventing STI at any age, but are user dependent and have high failure rates. Relying on oral emergency contraception is not recommended. Attendance for EC is a good time to discuss future contraception. You should advise doubling up with a more effective contraceptive method. Do not forget to discuss *Chlamydia* testing as prevalence is high in this age group.

No method is precluded by age, but it is important to elicit a careful clinical history in the form of medical, family, drug and smoking history and check blood pressure and BMI. Any findings that increase risk of CVD may mean avoidance of oestrogen-containing methods, particularly if there are multiple risk factors. However, in women with no risk factors, the COC has many health benefits.

DMPA contains progesterone only but is associated with amenorrhoea and decreased bone mass and may be unsuitable for some women. Other LARC methods such as the POI (3 years), IUD (10 years) and IUS (5 years) have the advantage of non-user-dependent compliance and rapid return of fertility on removal.

Less common methods such as diaphragms/caps and NFP may appeal to women wishing to avoid hormones because of medical conditions, drug regimes or past side-effects. Efficacy with these methods can be high, but they are very much user dependent. On its own, lactational amenorrhoea is a very effective method until weaning starts.

When childbearing is complete, many couples consider sterilization. Sterilization should be considered permanent and both methods carry intraoperative and postoperative risks. In modern society where partnerships commonly dissolve, LARC methods have the advantage of keeping fertility options open. Fertility declines from the age of 35 years but contraception is still required to avoid a late unwanted pregnancy.

KEY POINTS

- EC can be given up to 72 hours (3 days) after unprotected sex and in some cases up to 120 hours (5 days) after ovulation
- Oral EC needs to be taken as soon as possible to maximize its effectiveness
- Always offer an IUD as an EC option as it is >99% effective and can continue as contraception
- Prescribe a COC with the lowest VTE risk, even though the actual risk is very small
- The main advantage of the patch over the COC is compliance

- Swabs prior to IUD insertion and/or prophylactic antibiotics are only recommended if there is a risk of STI
- Sterilization under 30 years carries the highest regret and request for reversal
- Contraception is recommended for 2 years if menopausal before 50 years or for 1 year if a woman is over 50 years
- Any sex confers a risk of STI, offer testing at the same time as contraception

Further reading

The Faculty of Sexual and Reproductive Healthcare has published method specific guidance documents and ones for special groups that can be accessed through their website: http://www.fsrh.org/

Royal College of Obstetricians and Gynaecologists. *Male and Female Sterilisation: Guideline Summary*. Evidence based Clinical Guideline No 4, January 2004. [http://www.rcog.org.uk/resources/Public/pdf/Sterilisation_summary.PDF] Accessed 30 March 2008.

http://www.ffprhc.org.uk/admin/uploads/298UKMEC200506/pdf

Case 9 A 22-year-old woman presents with vaginal discharge

Morag is 22 years old and works in a grocery store. She has noticed in the last week or so that she has vaginal discharge. She has never had this before and she is worried about the colour and smell. She is too embarrassed to speak to her mother or her best friend. An article in her favourite magazine suggested that she get swabs taken at her GP clinic or local sexual health clinic.

What other information do you need?

Vaginal discharge is a common symptom with a number of different causes. Some are benign and some are potentially life-ruining or life-threatening. Formulating a differential diagnosis will help focus your line of questioning.

What is your differential diagnosis?

- Physiological
- Non-infective:
  - bacterial vaginosis (BV)
  - vulvovaginal candiasis (VVC)
- Sexually transmitted infection (STI)
  - *Chlamydia*
  - gonorrhoea
  - *Trichomonas vaginalis*
- Cervical lesions (ectopy, polyp)
- Foreign body

What further questions would help to pinpoint the diagnosis?
Physiological

Physiological discharge is the most common cause of discharge in women of reproductive age. However, it is a diagnosis of exclusion, meaning you have to exclude other causes first. The clue is that it is usually cyclical in nature.

Obstetrics and Gynaecology: Clinical Cases Uncovered.
By M. Cruickshank and A. Shetty. Published 2009 by Blackwell Publishing. ISBN 978-1-4051-8671-1.

Iatrogenic

You need to ask Morag about contraception. The combined oral contraceptive (COC) or the patch predispose to cervical ectopy. All contraceptive methods can give unpredictable bleeding which may be misconstrued as discharge. Intermenstrual bleeding is common with the intrauterine device.

Cervical ectopy

Ectopy is the physiological response to oestrogen. An ectopy is the appearance of the exposed glandular epithelium of the endocervix canal extending on to ectocervix (Plate 9.1). It is associated with increased oestrogen (puberty, pregnancy and taking exogenous oestrogen, e.g. COC). Mucous glands in the glandular epithelium produce increased discharge.

Bacterial vaginosis

BV is characterized by a grey discharge with a fishy smell. The use of vaginal douches or deodorants will predispose to BV by lowering the pH of the vagina.

Vulvovaginal candiasis

VVC is characterized by a thick white discharge and itching, redness and soreness of the vulva, vagina and anus. Pregnancy, diabetes and a recent history of antibiotics or steroid use can predispose.

Chlamydia, gonorrhoea and *Trichomonas*

You need to take a sexual history from Morag, specifically asking her about any episodes of unprotected sex. A history of a new sexual partner in the past 3 months or more than one partner in the past year increases the risk of STI. All three STIs can give symptoms of dysuria and dysparunia. *T. vaginalis* can cause soreness or itching in the genital area. A recent history of intermenstrual bleeding, breakthrough bleeding on contraception or postcoital bleeding would suggest *Chlamydia* or gonorrhoea. Remember to ask about symptoms associated with upper genital tract infection (pelvic pain, deep dysparunia).

Cervical polyp

Cervical polyps are usually asymptomatic but can cause intermenstrual or postcoital bleeding.

Foreign body

This is associated with offensive discharge. Ask specifically about tampon use and foreign body insertion.

Morag tells you that she uses 'the Pill' and tampons. She admits to only occasional condom use. She had thrush a couple of times in the past but her symptoms seem different and she has little in the way of itch. She has had five sexual partners in the past year and three of these were new partners. She has a vulval soreness but has not noticed any lumps. Sex has not been painful and she has no pelvic pain. She had her first smear about a year ago and the result was negative.

KEY POINT

You will not know the sexual history unless you specifically ask (Box 9.1). The questions are embarrassing but can be asked in a sensitive manner. The patient's response will guide you on what tests, advice and treatment are most appropriate.

Does she need to be examined?

Morag can be treated empirically for VVC or BV without an examination, if she gives a clinical and sexual history that is:
• Consistent with a non-infective cause for her discharge
• Low risk for STIs
• She has no symptoms indicative of upper genital tract infection
• She is able to return for follow-up if symptoms do not resolve

You should 'safety net' in these circumstances by saying if her symptoms do not settle or if they re-occur she should make an appointment for swabs. In this case, as her history is not typical of VVC or BV and she gives an increased risk of STI, she should be examined.

What should you look for on examination?

You need to inspect the vulva, perineum and anus for swelling, redness or fissures. You need to take note of any fishy or offensive smell.

Box 9.1 Example questions to elicit a female sexual history

Have you had any major health problems in the past?
Have you had any sexually transmitted infections in the past?
Have you ever injected drugs?
Have you a current or past sexual partner who has injected drugs?
Have you a current or past sexual partner who is HIV or viral hepatitis positive?
Have you a current or past sexual partner who is bisexual?
Have you a current or past sexual partner from outside the UK? If yes, which country?
Have you had medical treatment outside the UK? If yes, which country?
Have you had a non-professional body piercing or tattoo?
Have you had sexual contact with the commercial sex industry?
Have you ever been sexually assaulted?
Have you ever had an HIV test?
Have you had a new sexual partner in the past 3 months?
How many sexual partners have you had in the past 12 months? How many were new partners?

Regarding sexual contacts in the past 3–6 months, ask about
Date of contact
Name (if known)
Duration of contact
Sexual activity (e.g. oral, vaginal, anal, sex toys)
Condom use (never, sometimes, always)
Nationality

Speculum examination

You will see a cervical ectopy or polyp is present. There may be a lost condom, tampon or another foreign body. You will be able to view the discharge and assess its consistency and colour. As Morag has no upper genital tract symptoms, you do not need to perform a bimanual examination.

Morag does not have enlarged inguinal lymph nodes. Her vulva looks a bit red and swollen and you identify small warty lumps at the introitus. There is a definite fishy odour. On speculum examination she has a cervical ectopy. There is creamy discharge and the cervix looks inflamed.

What further investigations might help to distinguish the possible diagnoses?

• Assessment of vaginal pH using narrow range (pH 4–7) litmus paper is cheap and helpful if there is no onsite microscopy. Test secretions swabbed from the lateral vaginal walls. A pH ≥4.5 would suggest BV or *T. vaginalis* rather than VVC, but cannot distinguish between the two.

• A high vaginal swab (HVS) taken from the lateral and posterior vaginal fornices can be used for both dry and wet microscopy and direct bacteriological plating. This will test for BV, *T. vaginalis* and yeast.

• An endocervical swab to test for gonorrhoea.

• An endocervical swab will test for *Chlamydia*. This is usually a nucleic acid amplification test (NAAT).

• Some microbiology laboratories can test for both *Chlamydia* and gonorrhoea from the same sample so check with your local laboratory.

• Warts are a clinical diagnosis and a biopsy is rarely necessary.

> **KEY POINT**
>
> Take the gonorrhoea swab first as you want to sample discharge. Then take the *Chlamydia* swab as you want to collect cells as *Chlamydia* is an intracellular organism.

Morag's test results are shown in Fig. 9.1.

> **KEY POINT**
>
> If you are performing a test you must have consent and confirm how to contact the patient if their result comes back positive.

Can you now make a diagnosis?

Clinical examination of Morag confirms the presence of a cervical ectopy and vulval warts. Microbiological tests, reported 2 days later, confirm coexisting *Chlamydia* and BV.

Are these diagnoses expected?

A cervical ectopy is common in COC users. Genital warts and *Chlamydia* are common STIs in Morag's age group and Morag has put herself at risk of an STI by changing sexual partners and not practising safe sex.

```
Genital Specimen Investigation
Microscopy
  Pus cells +
  Gram negative bacilli +++
  Gram positive bacilli ++
  Epithelial cells ++
  T. vaginalis trophozoites Nil
  Film suggestive of Bacterial vaginosis
Culture
1 Profuse growth of Mixed Anaerobes


Chlamydia DNA test  POSITIVE
Please treat and refer to GU clinic
for contact tracing
-----------------------------------------------
Page: 1 u/k = Unknown        Sample Time: 9:30
Laboratory Number: 103456  Report Time: 12:19
Specimen: Endocervical swab
```

Figure 9.1 Morag's test results.

Many young women are embarrassed or frightened of intimate examinations. If Morag refused to be examined what could you do to aid the diagnosis?

You could ask Morag to take her own swab for BV, *T. vaginalis* and yeast. It might also pick up gonorrhoea, but an endocervical sample is more sensitive. For *Chlamydia* she could do a self-obtained low vaginal swab (SOLVS) or first void urine (FVU). An FVU sample is used as it provides a vulval wash with the highest bacterial load for DNA amplification. Patients need to be warned that repeat testing may be required if the result is indeterminate.

> **KEY POINT**
>
> Non-invasive tests are particularly useful if a patient is asymptomatic or does not need to or wish to be examined.

With diagnoses of cervical ectopy, genital warts, BV and *Chlamydia*, what treatment would you suggest?

Results usually take a few of days to process. If the history and examination point to a specific diagnosis, there is merit in starting treatment empirically. This is particularly relevant if the wait for laboratory confirmation could result in ascending infection to the upper genital tract. Upper tract infection is called pelvic inflammatory disease (PID) and the tubal damage can lead to ectopic pregnancy, tubal factor infertility and chronic pelvic pain.

> **KEY POINT**
>
> You should have a low threshold for empirical treating women at risk of STI.

Cervical ectopy

Cervical ectopy often does not need treating as the glandular epithelium will undergo metaplasia to squamous epithelium with time. In Morag's case, conservative management would be appropriate. If her discharge continues, you could offer cryocautery or suggest a change to a progesterone only method of contraception or a barrier method. However, she may not like the change and could risk an unplanned pregnancy.

Genital warts

This is an incidental finding. Treatment is for cosmetic reasons and aims to destroy the warts and assist the patient's immune system to stop producing more. Treatment options for warts include:

1 Freezing with liquid nitrogen.

2 Podophyllotoxin cream or solution is applied at home twice daily for 3 days per week.

3 Imiquimod cream is a non-specific immune system modulator. It is applied on alternate nights for a maximum of 16 weeks. It is expensive and except in the case of anal warts, should be used third line when previous treatments fail.

Bacterial vaginosis

This is not an infection but an overgrowth of the bacteria normally found in the vagina. This is why it is an '-osis' not an '-itis'. BV only needs treatment if the woman is symptomatic or pregnant. Treatment is usually with metronidazole either one dose (2 g) or twice daily dose (400 mg) for 5 days. Patients should not drink alcohol during treatment and for 24 hours after as it reacts with alcohol. BV is not an STI and partners do not need treatment. Recurrence is common.

Chlamydia

Chlamydia is an STI and treatment is a one-off dose of azithromycin (1 g).

Morag will be asked to abstain from sex for 1 week or until 1 week after her regular sexual partner has been treated. *Chlamydia* infections are asymptomatic in 50% and 70% of males and females, respectively. *Chlamydia* is most common in under-25-year-olds and those who do not use condoms.

Would your management be different if you thought Morag had an upper genital tract infection?

If she had upper genital tract symptoms (pelvic pain and/or dyspareunia) the diagnosis is PID and she needs a different course of antibiotics:

• Doxycycline 100 mg twice daily for 14 days and metronidazole 400 mg twice daily for 10 days

• If gonorrhoea is suspected or present, add ceftriaxone 250 mg IM once

Warn her about the side-effects of doxycycline – nausea on an empty stomach and photosensitivity (no sunbeds) – and the interaction between metronidazole and alcohol.

Morag is shocked to be told that she has two STIs and starts crying. She is devastated that her boyfriend has cheated on her.

What would you say to her?

Most patients find the diagnosis of STI distressing but it is better to know and be treated so that potentially life-ruining sequelae can be averted. These diagnoses do not confirm infidelity in her current relationship. In the case of genital warts, 70% of a sexually active population will have a genital human papilloma virus (HPV) infection at some stage, but only 1 in 5 develops warts. Because of its asymptomatic nature, she could have picked up *Chlamydia* from a previous sexual partner or her current partner may have brought it into the relationship from a previous partner.

You succeed in settling Morag down. Is there anything else you should discuss with her?

• Partner notification and health advisor support (Box 9.2)

• Information leaflets

• Safe sex

• Retesting for *Chlamydia*

Morag should ask her partner to attend a local genitourinary medicine (GUM) clinic or his GP for testing and treatment.

> **KEY POINT**
>
> To avoid reinfection, current sexual partner(s) should be tested and treated.

Box 9.2 Health advisor

The health advisor is specifically trained in partner notification. It is their job to identify potentially infected individuals and break the infection chain. They will trace contacts anonymously if the patient feels unable to do this. Ideally, they would see both Morag and her partner(s) individually and identify any other sexual partners from the past 3–6 months. This can be a difficult job as many index cases (positive patients) are too embarrassed to give names or do not know the name of casual sexual contacts.

At the GUM clinic, her partner's sexual history will be taken and he will undergo urethral swabs for *Chlamydia* and gonorrhoea or FVU for *Chlamydia*. He has about a 70% chance of being positive for *Chlamydia* and most GUM clinics would treat him empirically with azithromycin (1 g). The couple would be asked to abstain for 1 week. He would then see the health advisor for partner notification, information and support.

What safe sex advice do you give?

The best way to prevent STIs is to practice safe sex. This means using a condom for all untested sexual partners. Condoms should be used for oral, vaginal and anal sex. Non-penetrative sex (massage, masturbation) is safer. Most GUM and family planning clinics offer free condoms.

What about retesting?

Morag needs to be retested for *Chlamydia* at 3 or 6 months in case treatment has failed or she has a reinfection. It can be performed non-invasively using a SOLVS if the patient is asymptomatic.

KEY POINT

Retesting before 3 weeks will yield a false positive result as the amplification process will amplify dead chlamydial bacteria.

Morag agrees to speak to the health advisor on the telephone who agrees to contact Morag's other recent sexual partners as Morag does not have any contact.

Sexually transmitted infections commonly occur together. While gonorrhoea and *T. vaginalis* have been ruled out, there are other STIs that Morag may have contracted.

Which other STI tests might be recommended?

- HIV
- Syphilis
- Hepatitis B
- Hepatitis C

The decision to offer each test depends on Morag's sexual history (Fig. 9.1).

Morag is not keen on a HIV test as she does not consider herself to be in a high risk group.

HIV

It is estimated that 1 in 3 of those infected with HIV in the UK are unaware of their positive status. HIV is on the increase in the UK and the majority of diagnoses are in heterosexuals. Most heterosexual acquisition is from outside the UK, mostly Africa. Most UK acquired infections are in men who have sex with men. An HIV test is a blood test that looks for antibodies to HIV. There is up to a 3-month window period for the test as most people take approximately 6 weeks before developing antibodies. Patients may therefore have to return for a repeat test.

Syphilis

Most cases of syphilis occur in men who have sex with men (hence the question about bisexual partners in the sexual history) or in men who have had sex with someone who is from outside Europe. Syphilis is highly infectious during its second and third stage. Third stage or latent syphilis can cause gummatous syphilis, cardiovascular syphilis and neurosyphilis which result in serious damage to the heart, brain, bones and central nervous system. Routine testing is also carried out antenatally because of potential serious affects to the fetus. Testing is by a swab that collects a sample of fluid from any ulcer or, more commonly, by a blood test.

Hepatitis B

Hepatitis B is highly infectious, 100 times more so than HIV. Morag is at risk of hepatitis B because of her history of unprotected sex. You should ask about any risk factors that may increase her risk of contracting hepatitis B (Box 9.3). One in four carriers of hepatitis B develop severe liver disease leading to chronic hepatitis, cirrhosis and cancer. Hepatitis B is detected by a blood test looking for antibodies and you need to ask for hepatitis B core antibody on the request form.

Box 9.3 Risk factors for hepatitis B

- Intravenous drug use
- Current or past partner with hepatitis B
- Current or past bisexual partner
- Family relatives with hepatitis B
- Health care occupation
- Contacts with prison (self or partner)
- Travel or work in countries where virus is endemic such as South-East Asia, Middle and Far East, south Europe and Africa

Hepatitis C

Hepatitis C is rarely contracted through sex. The main risk factor is injecting drug use and it is estimated that 50–80% of past and current users are infected.

Is there anything else that could be offered to Morag in way of prevention?

Safe sex and the use of condoms have already been discussed with Morag. Another option is hepatitis B vaccination.

Morag's sexual history revealed multiple sexual partners in the past year but all from the UK. There was no history of injecting drug use or high risk partners. She had never been outside the UK, had never been sexually assaulted, and had only professional piercings and tattoos. She was deemed low risk for blood-borne virus infections, but testing for HIV and hepatitis B was recommended. These came back negative.

CASE REVIEW

This 22-year-old woman presented with the common complaint of vaginal discharge. A careful history, asking targeted questions, will help home in on a differential diagnosis. Most women of this age will be sexually active, meaning that iatrogenic contraceptive causes and STI infections should be high up on your diagnosis list. *Chlamydia* is found in 10% of sexually active 25-year-olds.

BV is a non-infective cause of vaginal discharge which is very common. Her symptoms were typical of BV and she could have started treatment for this on history alone. Normally, there should be a low threshold for performing a vaginal examination. In this case, taking genital swabs was useful as she was found to be *Chlamydia* positive. Most STIs, except genital warts and herpes, benefit from partner notification, testing and treatment.

A useful routine to follow is to take a HVS from the posterior and lateral fornices to test for yeasts, BV and *T. vaginalis*. Then take an endocervical swab for gonorrhoea and endocervical NAAT for *Chlamydia*. If she had refused examination, a self-obtained high vaginal swab and low vaginal NAAT swab could be collected. FVU is an alternative sample for *Chlamydia* testing. Evidence of her risky sexual behaviour gave an opportunity for education about safe sex, the offer of hepatitis B testing and vaccination, and the provision of free condoms.

KEY POINTS

- Women under 25 are often sexually active and this is a good opportunity to discuss both contraception and STI risk
- A sexual history is intrusive but can provide key information for the differential diagnosis, inform on appropriate testing and sampling sites, aid the partner notification process and focus education and prevention strategies
- There should be a low threshold to perform a vaginal examination if symptoms are present
- Always offer a chaperone for any intimate examination
- Swabs should include an HVS and two endocervical swabs

- If you are performing a test you must have consent and a means to contact the patient if their result comes back positive
- VVC and BV only need treatment if the patient is symptomatic and testing and treatment of male partners is not routinely recommended
- Partner notification is recommended for all STIs except genital warts and herpes
- Unprotected sex increases the risk of blood-borne viruses such as HIV, syphilis, hepatitis B and C
- Education, condom use and hepatitis B vaccination can reduce the risk of acquiring an STI

Further reading

Faculty of Family Planning and Reproductive Health Care Clinical Effectiveness Unit. FFPRHC and BASHH Guidance. The management of women of reproductive age attending non-genitourinary medicine settings complaining of vaginal discharge, January 2006 [http://www.fsrh.org/admin/ uploads/326_VaginalDischargeGuidance.PDF] Accessed April 2, 2008.

The British Association For Sexual Health website (www.bashh. org) has a comprehensive list of clinical effectiveness guidelines on all sexually transmitted infections, common presentations and other aspects of sexual health.

Case 10 A 29-year-old woman with an abnormal smear test

Christie Thomson is 29-year-old housewife. She is currently on maternity leave after the birth of her son Caleb 4 months ago. She had a normal delivery and initially breast fed but has changed to bottle feeding in the last 2 weeks. Her smear test was due 10 months previously but she postponed this as she was pregnant. She was well during her pregnancy and since delivery. She has not yet had a period.

She was reminded to make an appointment for a smear at her postnatal check and attended 3 weeks ago. The practice nurse said that her cervix looked normal so she was shocked when she received a letter to say that she had an abnormal smear result and that she would be sent an appointment to attend the colposcopy clinic at her local hospital. She has been worrying ever since and thinks that she may have cancer. Her maternal grandmother died from cervical cancer at age 48 and she knows her mother, who was a teenager at the time, found this difficult to cope with; she commented when Caleb was born how happy she was to have a grandson. Her mother urges her to find out when she will receive an appointment.

What should she do next?

The smear taker has the responsibility of informing women at the time they attend for screening of:

- The purpose of cervical screening
- The likelihood of an abnormal result
- What will happen if the result is abnormal

Women are often very anxious when they receive an abnormal smear result. Some women confuse cervical screening with a test for cancer (Box 10.1). If her local practice has not contacted her, she should get in touch to discuss her result. This may be by telephone.

Obstetrics and Gynaecology: Clinical Cases Uncovered.
By M. Cruickshank and A. Shetty. Published 2009 by Blackwell Publishing. ISBN 978-1-4051-8671-1.

Christie phones her practice and speaks on the telephone to the practice nurse who took her smear. She reassures Christie that the smear test shows only a mild abnormality and in other areas, she would be invited for a repeat smear in 6 months time as this may resolve spontaneously. However, local practice is to refer to colposcopy to look for precancerous changes. She is told that she should make an appointment for about 8 weeks' time.

Christie is very anxious about the delay. She is concerned that her smear was not taken when it had been due during her pregnancy and that her grandmother died from cervical cancer.

> ### KEY POINT
>
> It is safe and recommended practice to defer smears during pregnancy. The effects of pregnancy can make it more difficult to obtain an adequate specimen for cytology and woman often prefer to wait.

Christie receives an appointment for the colposcopy clinic and an information leaflet explaining what will happen at this appointment. She is confused about the grades of smear results and what this means for her.

What does Christie need to know about her smear result?

Different grades of dyskaryosis are associated with different levels of risk for underlying high grade cervical intraepithelial neoplasia (CIN) (Boxes 10.2 and 10.3). Borderline nuclear abnormalities (BNA) show no definite dyskaryosis and often regress. A repeat smear in 6 months is usually recommended. Women are referred for colposcopy if they have three consecutive borderline smears. Only 10% of women with persistent BNA smears will have underlying CIN.

Box 10.1 Human papillomavirus and natural history of cervical disease

As cervical cancer is caused by an oncogenic virus, human papillomavirus (HPV), it is not a familial cancer. There are over 100 different genotypes of HPV.

High risk HPV types (HPV 16 and 18) are oncogenic viruses. HPV DNA has been found in 99.7% cases of squamous cell cancer of the cervix. Remember HPV infection is common, with a lifetime incidence of 70–80%.

Women tend to acquire HPV infections around the time they start having intercourse. In most instances, HPV infection is transient; the woman's immune system effectively clears the virus and it has no clinical significance. Low grade cytological changes are often related to HPV infection (a small proportion being high risk types) rather than cervical intraepithelial neoplasia (CIN). In a small proportion of women, persistent HPV infection, in particular with high risk types, results in the development of high grade CIN (CIN 2 or 3). High grade CIN is premalignant in that, in a proportion cases, invasive cancer will develop in the subsequent 10–20 years. Low grade CIN (CIN 1), however, often resolves spontaneously. High grade CIN may not have a preceding low grade disease but both are HPV-related.

The NHS in the UK provides an HPV vaccination for girls aged 12–13 years against HPV 16 and 18.

Box 10.2 Dyskaryosis

This is a cytological term used to describe the nuclear changes in exfoliated cells picked up on the smear test. These include nuclear enlargement and irregularity in shape and outline of the nucleus. The grade of dyskaryosis is determined by the severity of these changes and also the increase in ratio of nuclear size to cytoplasm which is a reflection of the degree of loss of maturation of the cell; the higher the ratio the more severe the degree of dyskaryosis. The degree of dyskaryosis is not always reflected the degree of CIN in the underlying epithelium (Plates 10.1 and 10.2).

Christie's smear has shown mild dyskaryosis. In about 20%, there will be CIN 2/3 on colposcopy and biopsy. There are conflicting ideas on the management of low grade abnormal smears. Currently, some centres see women for colposcopy after a single mildly dyskaryotic smear to speed up the diagnosis of those with CIN. However, it is acceptable to repeat the smear in 6 months. Those women who still have an abnormal smear are then

---

Box 10.3 Cervical intraepithelial neoplasia

This is a histopathological term used to describe abnormal proliferation (dysplasia) of the squamous epithelium of the transformation zone of the cervix.

The grade of CIN relates to the proportion (in terms of thirds) of the epithelial thickness which has become dysplastic. Therefore, in CIN 3 there are full-thickness changes involving 3/3 of the epithelium. These changes are limited to the epithelium with the basement membrane intact. If the basement membrane is breached, this is invasive disease (cancer) (Plate 10.3).

---

sent for colposcopy. This allows some women to avoid unnecessary investigation.

Moderate or severe dyskaryosis (present in around 1.5% of smears) is associated with a 65–95% risk of having high grade CIN. This needs treatment to prevent progression to invasive cancer so surveillance is not offered (except during pregnancy).

What information should you elicit from Christie at the colposcopy clinic?

The aim of cervical screening is to reduce the risk of dying from cervical cancer by detecting and treating CIN. CIN is asymptomatic but it is common practice to ask specifically about symptoms associated with cervical cancer. These are intermenstrual bleeding, postcoital bleeding, postmenopausal bleeding and abnormal vaginal discharge.

You need to check the date of her last menstual period (LMP) and her method of contraception as biopsy and treatment should be avoided during pregnancy.

Remember, it is important to check that Christie understands the reason for her referral and what to expect at this visit.

Christie had some pink and brown discharge for 2–3 weeks after Caleb's birth but no bleeding since. She is not using contraception but has not yet had sex as she is too tired.

What would you look for on examination?

A speculum is inserted to view the cervix. Colposcopy allows magnification and good illumination of the cervix. The whole of the transformation zone needs to be identified. Initial examination allows the colposcopist to exclude any obvious signs of cancer. A weak acetic acid solution (3–5%) is applied directly to the cervix. This highlights areas of abnormality which turn white (acetowhitening) and capillary blood vessel patterns may be seen with high grade CIN. Acetowhitening can also be associated with active metaplasia of the transformation zone or human papillomavirus (HPV) infection. Following this, Lugol's iodine (aqueous iodine) can be applied. Normal squamous epithelium will stain brown (as it contains glycogen) but is not taken up by areas of CIN.

Christie's cervix looks normal (as she was told when her smear was taken) but CIN cannot be identified yet. On colposcopy, the whole of her transformation zone can be seen clearly. After applying 5% acetic acid, dense whitening of the epithelium with an obvious mosaic pattern of capillary vessels is seen (Plate 10.4). There are no bizarre or abnormal vessels which would suggest invasive disease. These findings are in keeping with CIN 3.

Can you now make a diagnosis?

Colposcopy will identify any area of abnormality. However, the histological diagnosis on biopsy is the gold standard for diagnosing cervical disease. Diagnostic biopsies are usually small punch biopsies (1–3 mm) and colposcopy allows the biopsy to be taken from the most abnormal area. Excisional forms of treatment (large loop excision of transformation zone [LLETZ]) also produce a specimen for histology.

What should you do next?

As Christie's initial referral smear was mild, there is a risk of treating unnecessarily if you treat her at this visit by LLETZ. She needs to have diagnostic punch biopsies taken to confirm the diagnosis.

The report from the pathology laboratory confirms the diagnosis of CIN 3 from her punch biopsies. Three weeks later, Christie receives a letter from the colposcopy clinic to advise her that her biopsies have confirmed precancerous cells (CIN) along with information regarding her treatment visit. She phones the clinic the make an appointment for treatment.

Treatment

Cervical treatments preserve reproductive function. This is important, as CIN is most prevalent in women age aged 27–33 years. Ablative or destructive treatments (cold coagulation, diathermy and laser ablation) destroy the transformation zone so a histological diagnosis is essential to confirm the presence of CIN and to exclude cancer before treatment. LLETZ is the most common mode of treatment. This procedure allows excision of the abnormal transformation zone using a diathermy loop and is usually performed under local anaesthetic in the outpatient clinic. Short-term side-effects are uncommon and include bleeding and infection. Cone biopsy is less common but it is an acceptable form of conservative treatment for microinvasive cancer (FIGO Stage 1a1).

On review, Christie has mild dyskaryosis identified as part of the national cervical screening programme. This was investigated by colposcopy and a diagnostic biopsy was taken targeted at the most abnormal area on colposcopy. Histology confirmed high grade CIN. High grade CIN is treated to avoid progression to invasive cancer over a 10–20 year period. As there is no evidence of invasive disease on her colposcopy examination or on punch biopsy, she can be safely treated using an ablative or excisional treatment.

Christie is relieved to be offered treatment promptly. She has a LLETZ procedure with a paracervical block using local anaesthetic and adrenaline to reduce bleeding. Following treatment, she had some period-like cramps for a day and some light vaginal bleeding for 3 weeks. She was advised to attend the colposcopy clinic in 6 months for a follow-up smear.

Follow-up

Follow-up following conservative treatment of CIN is important in the detection and early treatment of treatment failure or the development of recurrent CIN. Women who have been treated for high grade CIN have a relative risk for cervical cancer which is eight times greater than the general population. Follow-up with cervical smears is recommended after the treatment of high grade CIN (CIN 2/3) for 10 years in England and Wales and 5 years in Scotland. For low grade (CIN 1), annual follow-up is for 2 years across the UK. Colposcopy may be performed at the first follow-up visit 6 months after treatment but this is not essential. Once follow-up is completed women return to routine 3-yearly recall. Currently, there are HPV sentinel sites in England which use HPV testing to reduce the duration of follow-up.

CASE REVIEW

The cervical screening programmes in the UK have successfully reduced the incidence and mortality from cervical cancer. Women are identified and called for screening on the basis of age although the criteria vary across the UK. Mild dyskaryosis accounts for around 2% of all smear results and in a proportion of cases it is associated with high grade CIN. Colposcopy is used to illuminate and magnify the cervix to inspect the cervical epithelium and identify any areas suggestive of CIN and to exclude any obvious changes indicative of cancer.

Low grade CIN can be managed conservatively but can be treated in the same way as high grade CIN if it persists, if the patient requests treatment or if the woman has completed her family. Treatment of high grade CIN can be treated using ablative or excisional methods but the treatment success rate of around 95% is the same for all treatment modalities.

Women treated for CIN remain at an increased risk of developing cervical cancer compared to the general population so follow-up by cytology (or HPV testing in selected sites) is essential.

The impact of the HPV 16/18 vaccination programme for girls at age 12 years will take a number of years to be seen given the long natural history of HPV infection and the development of CIN and cancer.

KEY POINTS

- Cervical smear screening is aimed at detecting cytological abnormalities (dyskaryosis)
- Organized screening programmes have successfully reduced the incidence of cervical cancer
- The cervical sample taken uses a plastic broom sampling device and it is collected in liquid-based cytology medium. Although no longer a 'smear', may people still refer to cervical cytology samples as 'smear' tests
- Women are often very anxious on receiving an abnormal smear result or attending for colposcopy. It is essential to provide adequate information and support
- The investigation of these changes at colposcopy may identify premalignant disease (CIN)

- CIN is asymptomatic
- The diagnosis is made by histology of biopsies or treatment specimens
- This allows early treatment at its premalignant stage and prevention of deaths from cancer
- Treatment is usually LLETZ but ablative methods are also used
- Women should be appropriately counselled about the results of the smear and encouraged to attend follow-up investigation and long-term cytology follow-up

Further reading

NHS CSP document 20. *Programme management.* Sheffield, 2003.

Case 11 A retired schoolteacher presents with a feeling of 'something coming down'

Mrs Milne, a 63-year-old retired schoolteacher presents with a feeling of something coming down. She has noticed this is becoming more pronounced and sometimes she experiences an ache in the vagina, especially after a bout of constipation. She is now concerned because the lump is growing in her vagina and as a consequence she has abstained from intercourse with her husband. Mrs Milne knows a friend has similar symptoms, but she does not want to discuss such a personal issue with her. When she is requested to attend for a routine cervical smear, she asks the nurse for advice. The nurse suggests making an appointment with her GP.

What is the differential diagnosis?
- Prolapse of bladder, uterus or bowel
- Subcutaneous cysts in vagina or uterus wall
- Abscess within the vagina

What would you like find out from her history?
Presenting complaint
- Duration of feeling something coming down and any relieving or precipitating factors
- Urinary symptoms and duration:
  - dysuria
  - urinary frequency
  - incomplete emptying
  - manoeuvres to empty her bladder
  - nocturia
- Bowel symptoms and duration:
  - constipation
  - diarrhoea
  - any manual compression of vagina to empty rectum
- Vaginal discharge

- Sexual function:
  - pain on intercourse
  - obstruction on intercourse

Medical history
- Previous gynaecological surgery
- Connective tissue disorders
- Respiratory disease

Menstrual history
Age at menopause.

Obstetric history
- Parity
- Type of delivery
- Pregnancy or labour complications

Family history
Presence of connective tissue disorders.

Social
- Activities/job, such as heavy lifting, increasing pressure on pelvic floor
- Smoking

Drug history
- Steroids
- Anticlotting medication (e.g. aspirin, clopidogrel, warfarin)

Mrs Mine informs you her last period was 9 years ago and she has no bleeding since. She has always tended to be constipated, although she eats sensibly. She has no urinary incontinence, but she comments that after micturition she has had to stand and sit back on to the toilet to empty her bladder fully, especially if she has been on her feet all day. Since retirement, she enjoys hill walking, but her symptoms have put her off going out with her walking group because the lump causes discomfort the longer she stays on her feet.

Obstetrics and Gynaecology: Clinical Cases Uncovered. By M. Cruickshank and A. Shetty. Published 2009 by Blackwell Publishing. ISBN 978-1-4051-8671-1.

She has no previous surgery or connective tissue disorder (nor in her family) and is on no medication. However, she did have one child who was delivered by forceps 41 years ago and she had an extensive tear at the time which required several stitches.

What would you look for on physical examination?
General
Body mass index (BMI); obesity can increase the intra-abdominal pressure and precipitate prolapse. Evidence of smoking such as nicotine-stained fingers and hair may indicate respiratory problems.

Chest examination
Any respiratory disease should be assessed and can precipitate prolapse if persistent and long term, especially from bouts of coughing. Any untreated condition or smoking should be addressed in addition to the presenting complaint.

Abdominal examination
A pelvic mass (benign or malignant) can increase intra-abdominal pressure and cause pelvic floor descent. Any mass identified should be managed appropriately (see Case 12).

Pelvic examination
A bimanual examination will exclude any pelvic mass contributing to prolapse (Fig. 11.1).

The speculum examination enables staging of the prolapse (its anatomical severity) to be undertaken. There are several types of staging classifications, some involving the vaginal introitus, with others using the hymenal ring as the reference point. Using a Sims speculum enables parts of the vaginal wall which are descending to be retracted, allowing all aspects of the wall to be assessed. You need to ask the patient to cough to allow the true extent of descent to be identified. Sometimes both anterior and posterior vaginal walls are descending and two Sims specula can be used, or a sponge-holding

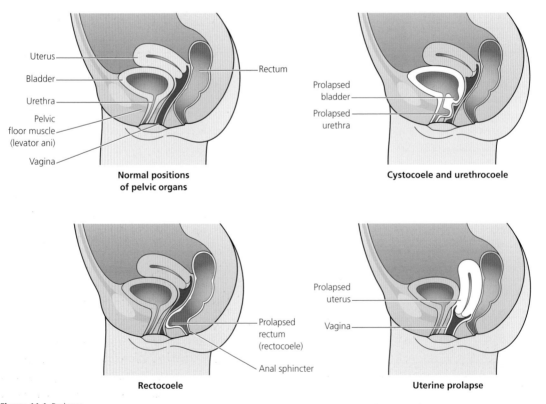

Figure 11.1 Prolapse.

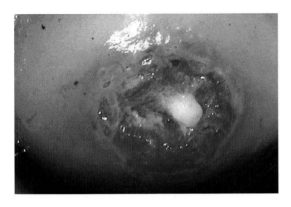

Plate 9.1 Cervical ectopy with mucous discharge.

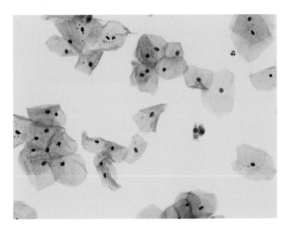

Plate 10.1 A cervical cytology sample with normal cells.

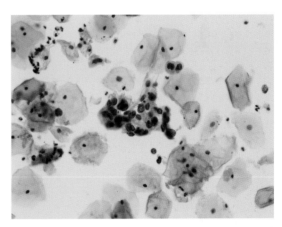

Plate 10.2 A cervical cytology sample with dyskaryotic cells.

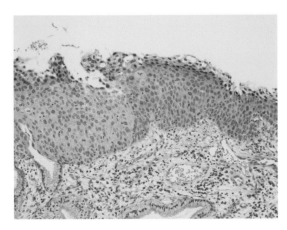

Plate 10.3 Cervical intraepithelial neoplasia 3 (CIN 3).

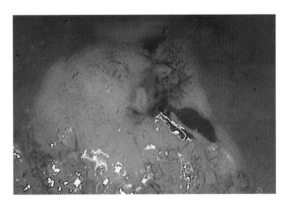

Plate 10.4 Colposcopic findings after the application of 5% acetic acid showing acetowhitening and mosaic and punctuation capillary vessel pattern.

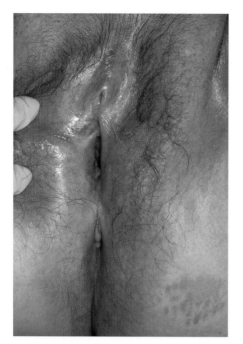

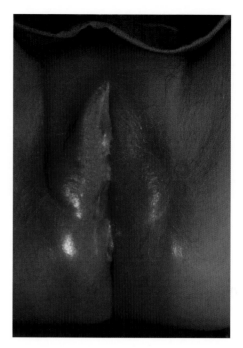

Plate 13.1 Vulual and peri-anal erythema and lichenification with loss of labia minora. Superficial ulceration on right side of fourchette.

Plate 13.2 Complete midline fusion from lichen sclerosus.

forceps (ovum forceps) to see the top of the vagina. You need to look for any uterine or vault descent (the middle compartment).

In patients who have had long-standing prolapse, trauma can occur on the exposed prolapsed area, sometimes in the form of an ulcer (decubitus). This can present with bleeding and the exposed cervix lying outside the vagina will be obvious on examination. It is important to check for incontinence of urine or faeces. Sometimes, urine will spontaneously expel on coughing at examination (stress incontinence). Sometimes, reduction of the prolapse precipitates incontinence. This may indicate distension of the prolapsed bladder with overflow incontinence. If faecal incontinence is present or has been suggested in the history, it may be appropriate to assess the anal sphincter by digital rectal examination.

Now review your findings so far

A 63-year-old woman presents with a 12-month history of a feeling of something coming down. She has given up her favourite pastime because of 'heaviness down below' and sometimes she has difficulty emptying her bladder. She is only slightly overweight, with a BMI of 28, is a non-smoker and has no medical problems. Abdominal examination has shown no mass, but on speculum examination the anterior vaginal wall descends 2 cm past the hymenal ring on coughing but is easily reducible on digital pressure. There is no presence of urinary or faecal incontinence or trauma on the exposed vaginal skin.

What other investigations would you recommend?

• *Mid-stream specimen of urine (MSSU).* If urinary symptoms are present, urine microscopy and culture should be performed
• *Urodynamic investigations.* Consider if stress urinary incontinence is identified
• *Surgical referral.* If there is faecal incontinence, referral to a colorectal surgeon as endoanal ultrasound and anorectal manometry may be required

What would you do next?

The most important action is to identify what the patient considers an acceptable management plan and how the prolapse affects her life. Not all prolapses require treatment and further questioning may be required as to the impact on lifestyle and any changes that can be made without further medical intervention.

Now review your differential diagnosis
Prolapse of bladder, uterus or bowel

The speculum examination has isolated the location of the prolapse to the anterior wall and thorough examination excludes concurrent descent elsewhere.

Sebaceous cyst or abscess in vaginal wall

Bimanual and speculum examination has excluded cysts in the vaginal wall or an abscess, which would be painful on palpation and possibly be discharging.

What treatment options would you offer?

1 *Conservative management.* As prolapse is not a life-threatening condition, further discussion should take place to identify an appropriate management plan. Sometimes all that is necessary is reassurance that this lump is not a cancer; however, in Mrs Milne's case, it has affected her quality of life and this should prompt you to discuss further management.
2 *Lifestyle factors.* You will have identified those likely to cause an increase in abdominal pressure in your history. These should be addressed, and you should give advice on weight loss and smoking as necessary.
3 *Pelvic floor exercises.* Exercises can successfully improve prolapse symptoms and also possibly improve surgical success if carried out preoperatively. These can be performed at home on a regular basis either with the tuition of a physiotherapist or a patient information leaflet. This type of management, however, does depend on the patient's commitment to undertaking their own treatment and continuing to perform them long term.
4 *Pessary.* For those who would prefer to have an instant 'fix', but not necessarily an operation, a pessary that elevates the prolapse can be an alternative. However, it is important to assess vaginal access and the dimension from the posterior fornix of the vagina to the pubis symphysis to identify the size of pessary that can be used. There are different shapes of pessary and the clinician's choice is dependent on the location of the prolapse. However, sometimes a pessary does not remain *in situ* and expels spontaneously, most notably when raised intra-abdominal pressure is present (such as defaecation).
5 *Surgery.* This is an option for patients who would prefer not to have a pessary and are found to have a prolapse sufficient to warrant surgery. The type of operation is very dependent on prolapse location and may involve the use of prosthetic material such as nylon mesh or biological grafts. Most prolapse surgery is performed

vaginally, but some techniques require abdominal access (either as minimal access or an open procedure via the abdomen). If surgical treatment is to be considered, biochemical renal and hepatic assessment as well as haematological indices are performed and checked pre-operatively. Elderly women and those with hypertension, respiratory or cardiac disease would also require a chest X-ray and electrocardiogram (ECG) for anaesthetic assessment. Prolapse surgery can be performed under regional block, e.g. spinal or epidural anaesthetic.

KEY POINT

Remember to stop any anticlotting agents 10 days before the operation to prevent intraoperative pelvic bleeding and to reduce the occurrence of intrathecal haemorrhage for those who have a regional anaesthetic for the operation. To compensate, most patients are given subcutaneous heparin pre- or postoperatively, dependent on what type of anaesthetic they have.

Mrs Milne decides to have a ring pessary inserted. She is assessed and a 71-mm diameter ring pessary is fitted comfortably. However, 4 days later, during a bowel movement, it falls into the toilet. She returns to the clinic and has a larger pessary inserted (81mm). She is seen for review 6 months later. Although the ring has remained in place, she has noticed some vaginal discharge and she is unhappy about having to attend for a ring change every 6 months. She thinks surgery would be a 'one-off' solution and asks to have 'the operation'. She has no risk factors for surgery or an anaesthetic and is admitted routinely. The operation consists of repairing the supporting tissues between the bladder and vaginal skin. She does not need a hysterectomy as she has no uterine prolapse.

Mrs Milne, after sufficient convalescence, is able to return to her hobby of hill walking and has no symptoms of prolapse. She understands the activities that could be detrimental to the repair of her prolapse given there is a 30% risk of failure with the operation. Mrs Milne performs her pelvic floor exercises daily to improve the postoperative success.

CASE REVIEW

This postmenopausal woman presented with a feeling of something coming down and urinary symptoms of incomplete emptying which impacted on her quality of life. She was primiparous having had a traumatic delivery but had no other factors impacting on her pelvic floor; she was only slightly above average BMI and did not smoke. Speculum examination indicated a cystocoele which descended beyond the hymenal ring on increased abdominal pressure, but this was easily reducible.

First line treatment was a ring pessary which was subsequently successful after appropriate sizing. However, Mrs Milne decided upon surgical management and continued to monitor her activities and promote success by continuing pelvic floor exercises.

KEY POINTS

- Any factor affecting abdominal pressure must be addressed in conjunction with any prolapse
- The anatomical site of the prolapse may affect the activity of pelvic organs such as the bladder and bowel
- Trauma can occur on the exposed prolapsed vaginal skin or cervix
- Pelvic floor exercises can successfully reduce symptoms and descent of prolapse but must be performed regularly to be effective
- Both type and size of pessary must be chosen appropriately for successful prolapse reduction
- Surgery has 30% failure rate
- The type of surgical procedure depends upon the prolapse and needs to be individualized

Case 12   A 57-year-old woman with abdominal swelling and vague abdominal pain

Mrs Rachel Simpson is a 57-year-old woman presenting with some abdominal swelling and vague abdominal pain. She noticed early in the year that she was putting on weight and her clothes were getting tighter round her waist. This was not unusual for her over Christmas and New Year but despite trying to diet, the swelling was now noticeable to her partner and a close friend had commented on it.

She is now very concerned as she finds she is unable to eat a full meal as she soon feels full up and uncomfortable. The same friend has long-standing irritable bowel syndrome and thinks Mrs Simpson has similar symptoms, especially the bloating. Mrs Simpson is very anxious as her brother died 10 years earlier from bowel cancer

What differential diagnoses immediately come to mind?
- Ovarian cyst
- Ovarian cancer
- Bowel cancer
- Ascites

What would you like to elicit from the history?
Presenting complaint
- Details of abdominal pain
- Gastrointestinal symptoms including constipation or other change in bowel habit, rectal bleeding or bloating
- Weight gain

Associated symptoms
- Symptoms of pressure on bladder (urinary frequency or incontinence)
- Symptoms associated with pressure on gastrointestinal tract (early satiety, reflux, heartburn)
- Symptoms of anaemia (tiredness)

Obstetrics and Gynaecology: Clinical Cases Uncovered.
By M. Cruickshank and A. Shetty. Published 2009 by Blackwell Publishing. ISBN 978-1-4051-8671-1.

Menstrual history
Age at menopause.

Obstetric history
Parity, type of deliveries and any complications.

Family history
History of cancer, particularly endometrial, colon or breast.

Mrs Simpson tells you that she thinks her last period was 7 years ago and she has had no bleeding since. She has no children and although she and her husband were investigated in her late twenties for primary infertility, no cause was found. She has had problems with constipation recently but no per rectum bleeding. She has been taking a laxative which she bought over-the-counter. However, this has aggravated the feeling of lower abdominal discomfort and made her feel generally unwell. There is no family history of endometrial or breast cancer but her brother was diagnosed with bowel cancer at age 62.

What would you look for on physical examination?
General examination
Pallor and cahexia are uncommon and even with advanced disease there may be little or nothing to find on general examination.

Abdominal examination
A distinct pelvic mass may be palpable above the pubic symphysis. The size of a mass arising from the pelvis is measured and stated relative to a pregnant uterus. A benign mass will tend to be well-defined, smooth and regular and may be mobile. A malignant mass will tend to be irregular, difficult to define and may be fixed. There may be abdominal spread and omental involvement may be detected as an irregular ill-defined mass in the upper or mid abdomen. There may be ascites causing distension with shifting dullness and a fluid thrill.

Pelvic examination

Bimanual examination. The uterus is likely to be small in a postmenopausal woman and can be felt separately but may become involved in a malignant mass. Feel on either side of the uterine body for adnexal masses. A malignant mass may be felt separately but may fill the pelvis giving an indistinct impression of thickening and induration.

> *To summarize your findings so far, Mrs Simpson is a 57-year-old para 0 + 0 with a 6-month history of increasing abdominal swelling and vague lower abdominal pain. On examination, her BMI is 28, and there are obvious abnormal findings, with generalized distension associated with shifting dullness and a fluid thrill. There is an irregular firm swelling in her upper abdomen which is difficult to define and nodular fixed mass in her lower abdomen. Pelvic examination is difficult as she is nulliparous and postmenopausal. She cannot tolerate a speculum and, on one finger vaginal examination, she has a craggy fixed mass which cannot be distinguished in origin.*

What do you do next?
Serum sample for CA125

Serum CA125 is often used in the investigation of women with a pelvic mass to identify ovarian cancer.

Ultrasound scan of her abdomen and pelvis

Ultrasound scan of the abdomen and pelvis will identify the mass. Important features that are suggestive of malignancy are used to calculate a risk of malignancy score (see below). These include the structure of the cyst in terms of cystic or solid, presence of ascites and disease beyond the pelvis.

What other investigations would you recommend?

• Full blood count (FBC) to check for iron deficiency anaemia
• Urea and electrolytes (U&E) to check renal function
• Liver function test (LFT) to check for evidence of liver involvement. Low albumin may be seen with ascites.

> *Her CA125 level is 437 IU/mL (upper limit of normal is 30 IU/mL) (Box 12.1).*
>
> *Her ultrasound report shows a slightly bulky uterus with a thin regular endometrium. Neither ovary can be identified separate to a large complex mass filling the pelvis. There are multiple locules and solid areas and there is free fluid in the abdomen.*
>
> *Her FBC, U&E and LFT are all within the normal range.*

Box 12.1 CA125

- Glycoprotein antigen
- Serum level raised in 80% of women with ovarian cancer but only 50% of women with stage I disease
- Used in detecting and monitoring epithelial ovarian tumours
- May also be raised with other malignancies (colon, pancreas, breast, lung)
- Also with benign conditions (menstruation, endometriosis, pelvic inflammatory disease, liver disease, recent surgery, effusions)

Table 12.1 Risk of Malignancy Index (RMI) scoring system.

Feature	RMI 2 score
Ultrasound findings: • Multiloculated cyst • Contains solid areas • Both ovaries involved • Ascites present • Intra-abdominal spread identified	0 = none 1 = Only 1 feature present 4 = ≥2 features present
Menopausal status	Premenopausal = 1 Postmenopausal = 4
CA125	IU/mL

What would you do next?
Risk of Malignancy Index scoring system

Risk of Malignancy Index (RMI) is used to calculate a score based on CA125 level, menopausal status and a score of the features identified on ultrasound. The score is used to predict the likelihood of an ovarian mass being malignant and appropriate referral for management (Table 12.1).

$$RMI = ultrasounds\ score \times menopausal\ score \times CA125(IU/mL)$$

KEY POINT

Women with an RMI score >200 should be referred to the gynaecology oncology service.

> **Box 12.2 Ovarian cancer and high risk groups**
>
> Only 5–10% of ovarian cancers are familial. High risk families for ovarian cancer have:
> - Two or more first degree relatives with ovarian cancer
> - One relative with ovarian cancer and one with breast cancer before age 50
> - One relative with ovarian cancer and two with breast cancer diagnosed before age 60
> - Known carrier of BRCA1 or BRCA2
> - Three or more family members with colon cancer, or two with colon and one with gastric, ovarian, endometrial, urinary tract or small bowel cancer in two generations
> - An individual with both primary ovarian and breast cancer

Now calculate the RMI (using RMI 2 score) for Mrs Simpson

$$Calculation\ of\ RMI = ultrasound\ score \times menopausal$$
$$score \times CA125(IU/mL)$$
$$4 \times 4 \times 37$$
$$\underline{6992}$$

Now review your differential diagnoses

1 *Ovarian cyst.* Unlikely because of her RMI score which greatly exceeds 200.

2 *Endometriomas.* These have a complex structure with solid elements and cause a modest rise in CA125 because of peritoneal involvement. This may be considered in premenopausal women but would not be expected as a new finding in a postmenopausal woman.

3 *Ovarian cancer.* This is the most likely cause so far based on her results and RMI score. No further imaging is required but you may consider a CT scan of her abdomen and pelvis for more information on the extent of metastatic disease such as omental involvement and peritoneal disease.

4 *Bowel cancer.* Although initially plausible, this is unlikely given the high risk of ovarian malignancy. However, the features of metastatic bowel cancer can be very similar to ovarian cancer and histology may be necessary to establish the diagnosis. She has a history of a first degree relative with bowel cancer but this does not put her at high risk of a genetic cause (Box 12.2).

5 *Ascites.* This has been found on her scan and is most likely caused by her advanced ovarian cancer and not a non-malignant cause. In uncertain cases, ascetic tap is performed for cytology and biochemistry.

What treatment options would you offer this patient?

The likelihood of malignancy and treatment plan needs to be discussed with Mrs Simpson. At this stage, she needs to be discussed at the gynaecology oncology multidisciplinary team meeting. The main stay of treatment is surgery and chemotherapy.

Surgery

Most women with ovarian cancer will require a laparotomy to establish the diagnosis, stage the extent of disease (Table 12.2) and to reduce the tumour bulk. Most women present with advanced disease (FIGO stage III or IV) and complete tumour clearance may not be possible. However, optimal debulking of tumour will improve the response to chemotherapy and prolong survival.

Laparotomy should include peritoneal cytology of any free fluid or washings, hysterectomy, bilateral salpingo-oophorectomy and omentectomy. The peritoneum, liver, spleen, appendix, retroperitoneal lymph nodes and the diaphragmatic surface need to be inspected or palpated for evidence of spread.

Mrs Simpson undergoes a laparotomy. She is found to have bilateral complex ovarian masses which are adherent to her uterus. Free fluid in her pelvis is aspirated and sent for cytology. Her omentum contains nodules of tumour and there are fine seedlings over her pelvic and abdominal peritoneum. Her liver and spleen are normal and there is no nodal enlargement in the pelvis or para-aortic nodes. A total abdominal hysterectomy, bilateral salpingo-oophorectomy and infracolic omentectomy are performed. At the end of the procedure the only residual disease is the 'sago seedlings' on her peritoneum.

Histology confirms a moderately differentiated serous cystadenocarcinoma of ovarian origin with involvement of the omentum. This is FIGO stage IIIc.

Chemotherapy

Women with disease other than FIGO stage Ia will require chemotherapy in addition to surgery (adjuvant chemotherapy). Chemotherapy should include a platinum agent in combination with paclitaxel or as a single agent if the patient is unfit or unwilling to have combination treatment. Mrs Simpson needs information on her likely response to chemotherapy and possible adverse

Table 12.2 FIGO (International Federation of Gynaecology and Obstetrics) staging of ovarian cancer and 5-year survival.

Stage	Findings	5-year survival
I	Confined to one or both ovaries	
Ia	Limited to a single ovary	90%
Ib	Limited to both ovaries	85%
Ic	One or both ovaries with surface tumour or ruptured capsule; malignant ascites or washings	80%
II	Extension to other pelvic structures	
IIa	Extension to uterus or tubes	70%
IIb	Extension to other pelvic tissues	64%
IIc	As IIa or but with surface tumour or ruptured capsule; malignant ascites or washings	
III	Peritoneal implants outside the pelvis or positive retroperitoneal nodes	
IIIa	Microscopic seedlings of peritoneum	59%
IIIb	Peritoneal implants <2 cm	40%
IIIc	Peritoneal implants >2 cm or positive retroperitoneal nodes	29%
IV	Distant metastasis including liver or pleural fluid	17%

effects when deciding on treatment. Cure is unlikely and the aim is to achieve remission from the disease.

Mrs Simpson decides on a combination of carboplatin and paclitaxel. She has six pulses of treatment. She is able to cope with the expected side-effects of nausea and vomiting with prophylactic antiemetics. She experiences complete hair loss during her treatment. At the end of her treatment, she has no clinical evidence of disease and her CA125 level has fallen to 10IU/L.

This is a complete clinical and biochemical response. However, she is likely to develop recurrence of her disease with in 6–36 months and is followed up in a multidisciplinary clinic. Follow-up provides reassurance and may identify recurrence. In the case of recurrence, chemotherapy may be used with the aim of palliating symptoms.

CASE REVIEW

This postmenopausal woman presents with increasing abdominal swelling and vague lower abdominal pain. The presenting symptoms of ovarian cancer are non-specific and there is no one typical symptom. However, her age, nulliparity and clinical findings of ascites and an irregular pelvic mass are very suggestive of ovarian cancer. Ovarian cancer is rare under the age of 30. The incidence increases with age, with peak prevalence in women in their fifties. Although this patient has a family history of bowel cancer in a first degree relative, this does not meet the criteria of a high risk family history.

The use of a RMI is useful in determining appropriate referral and is based on menopausal status, CA125 tumour marker level and ultrasound scan findings. Abdominal and pelvic ultrasound are the most important imaging investigations at this stage. As is often the case, ovarian cancer is often advanced before the patient presents with symptoms.

Epithelial tumours account for over 90% of all ovarian cancers and are usually associated with an increased CA125 although less often with FIGO stage I disease. Spread is often within the peritoneal cavity, and peritoneal and omental disease and ascites may be apparent on clinical examination or imaging.

First line treatment involves cytoreductive surgery with the aim of removing, or at least optimally debulking the tumour and chemotherapy. Optimal surgery will include a total abdominal hysterectomy, bilateral salpingo-oophorectomy and omentectomy. First line chemotherapy should be a combination of carboplatin and a taxane. Survival is related to the stage of disease at presentation. However, most women present with advanced disease when the 5-year survival is only 10–15% and most women will develop recurrent disease within 2 years.

KEY POINTS

- Pregnancy should be excluded in young women with a pelvic mass
- Benign pelvic masses such as benign ovarian cysts and fibroids are usually identified in premenopausal women
- Ovarian cancer should be considered in postmenopausal women with a pelvic mass
- CA125 and ultrasound are the most useful baseline investigations
- The aim of surgery is to make a diagnosis, stage the disease and to debulk the tumour as much as possible
- Except for very early stage disease (FIGO stage Ia), women will require combined chemotherapy

Case 13 A 68-year-old woman presents with long-standing vulval itch

Edith Catchpole is 68-year-old retired secretary. For the last 8 years, she has suffered from vulva itch. Sometimes the itch improves but it always flares up again. She cannot identify anything that triggers this. She has tried a number of different creams that she has bought from her local chemist. These are mostly thrush treatments and creams for 'personal itch'. She has been too embarrassed to see her GP. However, she can no longer cope as she often wakes up at night scratching, disrupting her sleep and making her skin painful. She feels that nothing really helps.

What are the most likely causes of itch for this patient?

Vulva itch, known as pruritus vulvae, is a common symptom which may be localized to the vulva or be part of a more generalized skin disorder. You need to consider likely causes in this age group with a long history and fluctuating course of itch:

- Lichen sclerosus
- Lichen planus
- Lichen simplex
- Vulval intraepithelial neoplasia (VIN)
- Vulval thrush

What further questions would help to establish the diagnosis?

You need to consider skin disorders and other relevant factors so you need to ask questions beyond a standard gynaecological history. You should ask about the following.

1 Other skin conditions that she has or has experienced in the past. The warm moist environment of the anogenital region means that the appearance may be atypical and not obviously recognized. For example, psoriasis in the vulva can appear as a well-demarcated, dark pink, moist area without the typical silver scale.

2 Her personal or family history of atopic conditions as well as any known allergies.

3 Her personal or family history of autoimmune disorders as some conditions (lichen sclerosus and lichen planus) are associated with autoimmunity. Ask about thyroid disorders, vitiligo, alopecia, diabetes and pernicious anaemia.

4 Any treatments she has tried so far (and their effects). You should specifically ask if she is using any over-the-counter preparations. She may even have tried treatments belonging to other family members or friends or ones purchased abroad. Topical treatments may aggregate the underlying condition or result in an allergic dermatitis.

5 Potential irritants including anything that comes in contact with vulval skin such as clothes, washing products (for herself and her clothes) and sanitary products.

Mrs Catchpole tells you that she has been using 0.1% hydrocortisone cream, prescribed by her GP, with some improvement in her symptoms. She also used a cream that she bought in a pharmacy in Spain which helped but she finished this some time ago. She has been washing with water only and using baby wipes to keep her vulva area clean. She wears white cotton underwear and uses blue-coloured toilet paper to match her bathroom suite. She sometimes wears panty liners when she goes out as she has occasional mild stress incontinence. She has an underactive thyroid gland. She has taken thyroxine daily for the last 10 years with no problems. She is on no other medication. She has no allergies and no other skin problems

Now review your list of possible causes
Lichen sclerosus

Lichen sclerosus can present at any age but is more commonly seen in postmenopausal women. It usually causes severe itching and soreness and most commonly affects

Obstetrics and Gynaecology: Clinical Cases Uncovered.
By M. Cruickshank and A. Shetty. Published 2009 by Blackwell Publishing. ISBN 978-1-4051-8671-1.

the vulval skin but it can be found in other non-genital sites. The whole vulva area and the skin around the anus may be affected. Uncontrollable scratching may cause bleeding and skin splitting and the skin becomes sore and tender.

Lichen sclerosus is not linked with female hormone changes, contraceptives, hormone replacement therapy (HRT) or the menopause. It appears to be an autoimmune condition, with around 40% of women with lichen sclerosus having or going on to develop another autoimmune condition.

Itch is related to active inflammation with erythema and keratinization of the vulval skin. Hyperkeratosis can be marked with thickened white skin. The skin can be fragile, classically demonstrating subepithelial haemorrhages (petechiae), and it may split easily. Typically, lichen sclerosus is seen around the introitus, perineum, labia minora, clitoral region and perianal skin. Continuing inflammation results in inflammatory adhesions. Often, there is lateral fusion of the labia minora which become adherent and eventual disappear. The hood of the clitoris and its lateral margins may fuse, burying the clitoris. Midline fusion can produce skin bridges at the fourchette and narrowing of the introitus. Occasionally, the labia minora fuse together medially which also restricts the vaginal opening and can cause difficulty with micturition and even urinary retention (Plate 13.1). Changes can vary in severity and features may be defined but are often diffuse. Some areas may be inflamed and red and others pale and crinkly or thickened and white. Lichen sclerosus does not extend into vaginal or anal mucosa.

Lichen planus

Lichen planus is a common skin condition that may affect the skin anywhere on the body. Lichen planus usually affects mucosal surfaces and is more commonly seen in oral mucosa. Typically, lichen planus presents with raised purplish plaques with a fine white reticular pattern (Wickham's striae). However, in the mouth and genital region it can be erosive and more commonly associated with pain rather than itch. Erosive lichen planus appears as well-demarcated glazed erythema around the introitus. The aetiology is unknown but it may be an autoimmune condition. It can affect all ages and does not seem linked to hormonal status.

Lichen simplex

Women with sensitive skin, dermatitis or eczema can present with vulva symptoms and these can result in

---

Box 13.1 Useful measures for vulval itch

Measures to improve vulval discomfort and irritation:
- Use a soap substitute to clean the vulval area. Water on its own tends to cause dry skin
- Shower rather than bath and clean the vulval area only once a day. Overcleaning can aggravate vulval symptoms
- Wear loose fitting silk or cotton underwear
- Sleep without underwear
- Avoid fabric conditioners and biological washing powders
- Avoid soaps, shower gel, scrubs, bubble baths, deodorants, baby wipes or douches in the vulval area
- Some over-the-counter creams including baby or nappy creams, herbal creams (e.g. tea tree oil or aloe vera) and 'thrush' treatments may include irritants
- Avoid wearing panty liners or sanitary towels on a regular basis
- Avoid antiseptic (as a cream or added to bath water) in the vulval area
- Wear white or light coloured underwear. Dark textile dyes (black, navy) can irritate sensitive skin
- Use white toilet paper

---

lichen simplex, a common inflammatory skin disease. It presents with severe itch, especially at night, and is caused by prolonged inflammation and scratching which thickens the skin. This is usually triggered by a chemical dermatitis but is sometimes linked to stress or low body iron stores.

Specific allergic reactions can be found in the vulva area from common allergens including perfumes, preservatives in topical treatments, rubber and textile dyes. Washing powder, fabric conditioners, sanitary towels or panty liners and synthetic underwear may be irritants. Most women with a vulva disorder will benefit from advice on general care of vulval skin and avoiding potential irritants (Box 13.1).

Vulva intraepithelial neoplasia

VIN is an uncommon premalignant condition of the vulva skin with a similar natural history to cervical intraepithelial neoplasia (CIN). Six per cent of women with CIN (see Case 10) will also have VIN. However, not all VIN is human papillomavirus (HPV) related, particularly in older women. HPV-related VIN is more common in younger women. Without treatment, approximately 40–60% of cases will progress to cancer. The itch is intractable although the use of emollients may help. It appears as raised papules or plaques which can look warty. It may be erythematous, white/keratotic or pigmented. Common sites are periclitoral, labia minora and perineum. It can extend to perianal skin and it may also be associated with vaginal intraepithelial neoplasia.

Vulval thrush

Vaginal thrush, characterized by a thick white discharge, is more common than vulval thrush. With an anogenital infection, irritation and soreness of the vulva and anus are more likely and it is not associated with chronic itch in postmenopausal women. Diabetes, obesity and antibiotic use may be associated. Vulval candidiasis may become chronic and is more likely to present like intertrigo with a leading edge of inflammation extending out from the labia majora to the inner thighs. Prolonged topical antifungal therapy may be necessary to clear a skin infection and advice on general care of the vulva may reduce the predisposition to this condition.

Do you need to ask any more specific questions?

Women may not volunteer information about sexual function but this can be a distressing aspect of vulva disorders.

> *On questioning, Mrs Catchpole says that she lives with her 79-year-old husband. They have not had penetrative sex for the last 2 years as she is too sore and attempts at sex resulted in skin splitting at the entrance to her vagina with pain and some bleeding. She tells you that her husband is very patient and although she is not particularly interested, she misses the intimacy and knows that her husband would like to resume a sexual relationship.*

KEY POINT

Vulva conditions often impact on sexual function and you may need to ask specifically, especially in older women.

What would you look for on examination?

General examination

Vulva symptoms may be the presenting feature of generalized skin disorders. You should look at common sites for eczema, psoriasis, dermatitis and intertrigo including hands, flexor and extensor aspects of joints, hairline including behind ears, submammary and waist areas.

Genital examination

Many causes of vulval itch can be identified by examination of the external genitalia. It is important to examine the vulva systematically with adequate light and exposure. This is best using a good light source with the patient on an examination couch with legs raised into a modified lithotomy position. Colposcopy is not necessary. You need to check labia majora, both sides of the labia minora and clitoral hood, the fourchette, perineum, perianal skin and natal cleft. It can be useful to use two cotton buds to move skin folds to ensure complete inspection.

If there is no obvious abnormality, you should ask the patient to identify the symptomatic area. However, in lithotomy position, a few women struggle to identify the area themselves and some women may never self-examine or be familiar with their vulva anatomy.

Speculum examination

There is no indication to perform a speculum examination as she has no vaginal symptoms. If she had features of VIN, it would be important to examine other lower genital tract sites including the vagina and cervix.

What further investigations might help to distinguish the possible diagnoses?

You may want to confirm the diagnosis by biopsy. This is not necessary unless you suspect VIN which must be diagnosed histologically and invasion needs to be excluded. You may reconsider biopsying if the diagnosis is not obvious or at a later date if the patient does not respond to treatment.

Let us review the examination findings

On examination, there is no evidence of skin disease at non-genital sites. There are obvious areas of erythema and pale crinkly skin which extends to the perianal area. Both labia minora appear to be absent and the clitoris not clearly defined. There are some telangectasia and a small area of ulceration (Plate 13.2).

Do you need to take a biopsy?

The history and examination findings suggest a diagnosis of lichen sclerosus. However, if you are suspicious of the area of ulceration, you may want to take a biopsy (Box 13.2).

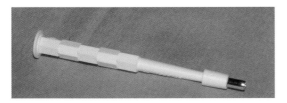

Figure 13.1 A Keyes punch.

> **Box 13.2 Vulval skin biopsy**
>
> Small diagnostic biopsies can be taken in the clinic under local anaesthetic. A Keyes punch (Fig. 13.1) will produce an adequate sample and avoiding crushing the tissue. You can control any bleeding by pressure, silver nitrate pencil or a undyed absorbable suture

---

The skin biopsy shows epidermal thinning, hydropic degeneration of basal cells, hyalinization of the dermis and subdermal lymphocyte infiltrate. Inflammatory changes are seen in all zones of the skin but in particular there is a band of inflammation in the dermis. These features support the clinical impression of lichen sclerosus.

Can you now make a diagnosis?

These findings confirm your history and your clinical examination findings.

Management

The main treatment is a prolonged course of ultra-potent steroid cream. This is applied once daily to the whole affected area for a month and then gradually reduced. With lichen sclerosus, topical steroids should reduce the itching quite quickly and any skin splits should begin to heal. Loss of normal vulval architecture will not alter and skin colour changes may not return to normal. Lichen sclerosus is a lifelong condition but treatment and lifestyle changes can control symptoms very well.

> **KEY POINT**
>
> Remember to discuss side-effects from steroids. Although this can be a problem with oral steroids, skin thinning is uncommon if a reducing regime is used to avoid excessive use.

An important part of the treatment is general care of the vulval skin and avoidance of any potential irritants that may worsen vulval irritation (Box 13.1).

Follow-up

You see Edith in 4 months' time for review. She has followed the reducing regime for the topical steroid cream and is now using it once a week. She is delighted that her itch and irritation have completely resolved. She continues to use an emollient daily and soap substitute to wash in the shower. However, she says that the skin still feels tight and she is still unable to have sex.

On examination, the condition of her vulva skin is very good with resolution of the erythema and hyperkeratosis. However, the introital narrowing and reabsorption of her labia minora remain unchanged.

Can you do anything to resolve her aparunia?

Surgery may be offered if the lichen sclerosus has narrowed the vaginal opening so that it obstructs micturition or penetrative sex. This may require a Z-plasty or local skin flaps to release scarring. Surgery itself will not cure lichen sclerosus and it is important to have any active inflammation controlled before surgery.

> *Edith decides that she does not want to undergo surgery and will continue to use emollients and her steroid cream when required to control any recurrence of her symptoms.*

Does she require any further review?

There is a 4% lifetime risk of developing squamous cell cancer of the vulva in the skin affected by lichen sclerosus. Edith needs to have information on this risk and to know to report any ulcers or lumps that do not respond to topical steroids.

CASE REVIEW

Vulval itch is a very common complaint and most women will initially self-medicate. It is often self-limiting but chronic vulval itch suggests an underlying vulval dermatosis or dermatitis secondary to use of potential irritants or overcleaning the vulva area. History-taking and examination of the skin are fundamental to making a diagnosis. Swabs should be taken if you suspect vulval thrush or a superadded infection. Biopsies are not always necessary unless you suspect VIN or invasive disease or if the condition does not respond to treatment. General care of vulva skin and avoidance of potential irritants benefits most conditions.

Lichen sclerosus is a chronic inflammatory skin which is often seen in postmenopausal women. The incidence appears to be in the order of 1 in 300–1000 of female adults and children. There may be an autoimmune basis to the development of lichen sclerosus. Over 20% of affected women have one or more first degree relatives with auto-immune-related disorders. Alopecia and vitiligo are the most commonly associated disorders but thyroid disease, pernicious anaemia and diabetes mellitus are also seen.

The main symptom is severe itch but it also causes discomfort, pain and dysparunia. There is often distortion or loss of the normal vulval architecture with labia minora or clitoral fusion and introital narrowing. The skin can easily split or tear. Many women find the symptoms embarrassing and distressing and have concerns about sexual function.

The typical clinical appearance is pale atrophic wrinkled skin, leucoplakia, telangectasia and erosions which form a figure of eight distribution around the vulval and anal areas. The symptoms often follow a fluctuating course with episodes of reactivation.

The main aim of therapy is to achieve good symptom control with the use of ultra-potent topical steroids and general care of the vulva. However, anatomical damage cannot be reversed. Surgery is limited to relieving symptoms secondary to labia fusion or introital narrowing. The risk of squamous cell carcinoma is about 4%.

KEY POINTS

- Vulval itch is a very common complaint
- The history required for vulval skin disorders differs from a standard gynaecological history as you need to know about other skin disorders and related factors
- You need to ensure good positioning of the patient and a good light source and take a systematic approach to examining the anogenital region
- Skin biopsy is not always necessary unless you suspect malignant disease or the condition does not improve in response to first line therapy
- Advice on general care of vulval skin and avoiding irritants often benefits women with vulval skin disorders in addition to specific therapies

- Lichen sclerosus is a life-long condition but good symptom control and prevention of tissue destruction can be achieved with ultra-potent topical steroids
- Lichen sclerosus is associated with a 4% risk of squamous cell cancer of the vulva and women need to know the signs or symptoms to look out for
- Surgery is rarely required for lichen sclerosus except to correct the effects of scarring such as aparunia or urinary retention

Case 14 A 30-year-old woman with a postdated pregnancy

Mrs Timmons is a 30-year-old woman in her first pregnancy. It has been an uncomplicated pregnancy but her baby was due 7 days ago and she comes to the antenatal clinic to discuss what to do.

What should happen at the clinic?

• Routine antenatal assessment: blood pressure (BP) and urinalysis
• Abdominal examination including symphysiofundal height (SFH), presentation of fetus and auscultation of fetal heart
• Enquire about general well-being and fetal movements

She tells you that she feels tired but well. She has been feeling plenty of normal movements from the baby. Her blood pressure is 120/80 mmHg which is normal for her and her urinalysis is negative. Her baby feels well grown (SFH is 39 cm), is in a cephalic presentation and the fetal heart is clearly heard. She asks you when you might induce her labour.

What do you say?

This seems to be a 'low risk' pregnancy and therefore national guidelines suggest induction of labour between 41 and 42 weeks. This maximizes the rate of spontaneous labour, decreases perinatal mortality resulting from postmaturity but does not increase the caesarean section rate from failed induction of labour.

She may wish to have a vaginal examination and membrane sweep as there is good evidence that this increases the spontaneous labour rate in postdated pregnancies. Performing a membrane sweep increases the discomfort of the examination and often causes a small amount of bleeding.

Obstetrics and Gynaecology: Clinical Cases Uncovered.
By M. Cruickshank and A. Shetty. Published 2009 by Blackwell Publishing. ISBN 978-1-4051-8671-1.

What will you tell her about your vaginal examination findings?

When a vaginal examination is performed before labour the findings are, by convention, assigned a score known as a Bishop's score which gives information about the favourability of the cervix in relation to labour (Table 14.1).

She accepts a vaginal examination and membrane sweep. Her Bishop's score is 5 and you book a date for induction at term +10. She asks you what will happen when she attends for induction.

What information would you discuss with her?

She will be admitted to an antenatal ward. The baby's heart rate will be monitored using cardiotocography (CTG) to ensure the baby is well. She will have a vaginal examination and prostaglandin (PGE$_2$) tablets will be inserted into the vagina. These tablets soften and shorten the cervix in preparation for labour.

If she is not labouring she will be given another dose of prostaglandins after 6–8 hours. A maximum of 6 mg PGE$_2$ tablets will be used. If she does not labour she will have her waters broken (amniotomy) and be started on oxytocin to stimulate her contractions.

She understands and is happy with this plan. At 23.30 that evening she calls the labour ward to say she thinks she is having contractions.

What questions will you ask her?

• When did the contractions start?
• How often are they coming and how long do they last?
• Does she have any vaginal bleeding or discharge?
• Does she think her waters have broken?
• Is she feeling the baby moving?
• Has she tried anything for the pain and is she still coping at home?

Mrs Timmons says she has been having pains roughly every 10 minutes since she went home from the antenatal clinic but now they are coming every 5 minutes. She thinks they last about 1 minute. She had paracetamol earlier but is not coping well with the pains now. She has no vaginal bleeding or discharge and the baby is moving normally. She is keen to come to hospital. You advise her to come to the labour ward.

What will you do when she arrives?

- Perform a CTG
- Assess the contractions for timing and duration
- Perform abdominal and vaginal examinations

She arrives at 00.30. She looks sore and seems to be contracting 3:10 minutes. The CTG is reassuring. Examination reveals that the baby is in a cephalic presentation. Vaginal examination shows that the cervix is 5 cm dilated and fully effaced. The vertex of the fetal head is 1 cm above the ischial spines (Vx 0–1) and the position of the fetal head is thought to be occipito-posterior.

What will be the plan for Mrs Timmons' labour?

- Adequate analgesia
- Intermittent auscultation of the fetal heart
- Repeat vaginal examination in 4 hours to ensure progress

Mrs Timmons has intramuscular morphine for pain. The fetal heart rate remains reassuring and she is reassessed after 4 hours. Unfortunately, she is still 5 cm dilated. Since the morphine her contractions have decreased to 1:10 minutes (Fig. 14.1; Box 14.1).

Table 14.1 Bishop's score. A Bishop's score <7 is considered unfavourable and usually indicates a more difficult induction process. Scores ≥7 indicate a favourable cervix.

Cervical feature	Score			
	0	1	2	3
Dilatation (cm)	<1	1–2	2–4	>4
Length (cm)	>4	2–4	1–2	<1
Consistency	Firm	Average	Soft	–
Station	−3	−2	−1/0	+1 +2
Position	Posterior	Mid/anterior	–	–

Box 14.1 The partogram

The partogram is a graphical representation of progress in labour and of maternal and fetal observations. The excerpt in Fig. 14.1 only shows cervical dilatation but in reality it charts maternal pulse, BP and temperature every 15 minutes. Fetal heart rate is also noted every 15 minutes. Frequency and strength of uterine activity is recorded every 30 minutes as is the colour of any liquor draining and any drugs administered. Cervical dilatation, and descent and position of the fetal head are marked down after each vaginal examination.

The partogram therefore provides an 'at a glance' guide to the progress of labour and the maternal and fetal condition.

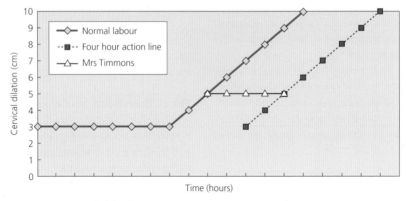

Figure 14.1 Partogram to assess progress in labour.

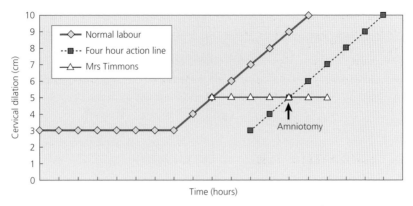

Figure 14.2 Partogram to illustrate slow progress in labour.

What is the plan now?

Perform an amniotomy to attempt to improve the uterine activity. Reassess in 2 hours to ensure progress.

> An amniotomy is performed and the liquor is clear. Mrs Timmons' contractions remain 1:10 minutes and she is able to sleep on and off during the next 2 hours. She is reassessed at 06.30 and found to be 5 cm dilated and the baby is felt to be still occipito-posterior (Fig. 14.2).

What will you tell Mrs Timmons?

Her progress in labour is slower than would be expected. This is probably because her contractions are suboptimal (we would aim for 4–5 moderate to strong contractions in 10 minutes). The baby's head is in a malposition (occipito-posterior) which makes labour less efficient (Box 14.2).

What intervention would you recommend?

As her uterine activity is now virtually non-existent, augmentation of her labour with oxytocin is recommended and reassessment of cervical progress 4 hours after good contractions.

> She accepts augmentation of her labour. She is commenced on a CTG which is reassuring and oxytocin is commenced. The oxytocin is gradually escalated and 90 minutes later she is contracting well with four moderate contractions in 10 minutes. She is now very sore and requests an epidural.

What information should you give her?

The anaesthetist will explain the procedure to her and make sure she understands it. She will then be asked to

---

Box 14.2 Progress in normal labour

Active labour is diagnosed in the presence of painful regular uterine activity once the cervix has reached 4 cm dilated and is fully effaced. In 1955, Friedman studied 200 normal women and determined that the slowest 10% progressed at 1 cm/hour in the active phase of labour. These figures are extremely small and were taken a long time ago and since then mothers and babies have changed significantly. Additionally, these data have not been replicated in other trials and the recent NICE guideline on intrapartum care recommends using 2 cm/4 hours as the minimum acceptable progress in the active first stage of labour. NICE apply this definition of delay in first stage to either primigravid or parous women. However, it should be borne in mind that labours in multiparous women are usually significantly faster than in primigravidae and if they are progressing slowly this should alert the attendants to the fact that something may be wrong. The WHO recommend a 4-hour action line on the partogram which indicates when labour is progressing at a rate 4 hours more slowly than expected. If this line is crossed once active labour is diagnosed, some action should be taken to accelerate or end labour in order to minimize risk to mother and baby.

---

either lie on her side or sit up and curve her back out. The anaesthetist will put some local anaesthetic in the skin and muscle of her back and then put a needle in her back to find the epidural space. A fine flexible tube is pushed through this needle, the needle is then removed. Drugs (local anaesthetic and analgesics) are given through the tube which is known as a catheter.

The epidural usually works within 10–20 minutes. It remains in place until after she has delivered her baby. A

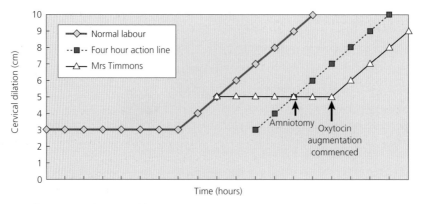

Figure 14.3 Partogram illustrating good progress with oxytocin augmentation.

measured amount of drugs may be given each hour or her epidural may be topped up using a syringe. Occasionally, epidurals do not give good pain relief. If this happens the epidural may need to be repositioned, a different combination of drugs used or the epidural may need to be replaced.

Advantages of an epidural
• Epidurals nearly always give good pain relief
• Because the drugs used are injected into the women's back, very little goes through to the baby

Disadvantages of an epidural
• The woman's blood pressure may drop, which can make her feel sick and dizzy. If this happens she will be asked to turn onto her side, she may be given fluid through a drip and might possibly need an injection to bring her blood pressure up again.
• Her mobility is likely to be limited.
• She may not be able to pass urine. If this happens a catheter will be used to empty her bladder.
• She may feel itchy; sometimes the combinations of drugs used can be altered to help relieve this.
• A small number (about 1%) of women develop a severe headache following an epidural (dural puncture headache). This can usually be effectively treated fairly quickly, but it can sometimes last for a number of weeks.
• She may develop a high temperature which could lead to an abnormally fast heart rate in the baby. This may lead to her and/or her baby being treated with antibiotics and screened for infection.
• There is an increased risk of the baby being delivered by forceps or ventouse.

She is seen by the anaethetist and her epidural is sited. It works well and there are no further problems until she is reassessed at midday as planned. Her cervix is now 9 cm dilated and the baby has turned to a much more favourable occipito-anterior position, it has also descended through the pelvis and the fetal head is now 1 cm below the ischial spines (Fig. 14.3).

What is the plan now?
She has made good progress since she was commenced on oxytocin so labour should be allowed to continue normally. Continue oxytocin and reassess in 1 hour when it is expected that she will be fully dilated.

She is reassessed after another hour and is fully dilated; the CTG remains reassuring. The plan is to allow a further hour for descent of the fetal head and then allow active pushing to try to effect delivery. Mrs Timmons is happy with this plan.

You are called to see her 2 hours later when she has been pushing for 1 hour but the baby is not delivered (Box 14.3).

What factors are important in deciding what to do?
Maternal factors
• Is she well? Are her pulse, BP and temperature all normal?
• Is she comfortable with her epidural?
• Have the contractions remained good and is she pushing well?
• What does she want to do?

Box 14.3 Second stage of labour

NICE guidelines divide second stage into a passive and an active phase. Passive second stage of labour is defined as the finding of full dilatation of the cervix prior to or in the absence of involuntary expulsive contractions. The active second stage of labour commences at full dilatation when the baby is visible, there are expulsive contractions or other signs of full dilatation or active maternal effort is commenced in the absence of expulsive contractions (most commonly in the presence of epidural analgesia). Delivery will usually have occurred after 3 hours of active second stage in primigravidae and after 2 hours in parous women. To allow for delivery within these time frames it is recommended that referral regarding delay in second stage be made to medical staff after 2 hours in primigravidae and 1 hour in parous women.

Fetal factors

- Is the CTG reassuring?
- Is the vertex advancing?
- What are the findings on vaginal examination?

Mrs Timmons' observations are all normal, she is comfortable and she has been pushing well with good contractions but she is exhausted and keen for the baby to be delivered. The CTG shows a few early decelerations but is otherwise reassuring for second stage labour. The vertex was advancing and is just visible at the height of the contractions but has not moved much in the last 20 minutes.

There is no head palpable in the maternal abdomen and vaginal examination confirms that the cervix is fully dilated, the fetal head is in an occipito-anterior position and it is at the ischial spines plus 2 cm (Vx 0 + 2).

What will you tell her now?

The options are assisted vaginal delivery or to continue actively pushing to try for a spontaneous vertex delivery. It should be quite safe to deliver the baby with forceps or a ventouse in the delivery room if she wishes.

I *Mrs Timmons agrees to assisted vaginal delivery.*

What preparations are required to deliver the baby?

The anaesthetist should be called to top up her epidural for delivery. Mrs Timmons should have her legs placed in the lithotomy position. She should have the vulva cleaned and draped and the bladder should be emptied using an in–out catheter.

The forceps or ventouse should be applied with contractions and the position of the instrument needs to be checked. Traction should then be applied with contractions until the head is crowning and then a right medio-lateral episiotomy should be made to protect against third or fourth degree perineal tears.

Once the head is delivered the instrument should be removed to allow the head to restitute prior to delivery of the baby's body. Once the baby is delivered, the placenta can be delivered by continuous cord traction and the episiotomy repaired.

She delivers a male baby weighing 3.45 kg in good condition by ventouse. The episiotomy is repaired and her total estimated blood loss is 350 mL. Mrs Timmons is very happy with the outcome and will be fit for discharge in a day or two.

CASE REVIEW

Mrs Timmons, a 30-year-old primigravida with an uncomplicated antenatal course, was due to be induced at T + 10 days for the indication of postdates. She had a membrane sweep some days prior to the planned induction and actually went into labour spontaneously before her date for induction. Progress in labour was slow, and augmentation was performed initially with an artifical rupture of membrances and then an oxytocin infusion. She had morphine and followed by an epidural for pain relief. She reached full cervical dilatation and after allowing time for the head to descend, she commenced active pushing. However, delivery did not occur spontaneously and an instrumental delivery was successfully performed for the indication of maternal exhaustion and prolonged second stage.

Slow progress is common in labour, especially in primigravidas. Except in highly multiparous women or those with previous caesarean sections when augmentation in labour is relatively contraindicated, labour can be augmented with oxytocin-like compounds to try to achieve a vaginal delivery providing there are no concerns about maternal or fetal well-being.

Augmenting labour in this way will reduce the numbers of caesarean sections performed for lack of progress. It is necessary to monitor both mother and baby carefully during this process as oxytocin augmentation carries some additional risks to both, over and above normal labour. Continuous fetal heart rate monitoring (CTG) is required because of the risk of fetal distress secondary to uterine hyperstimulation.

Assisted vaginal delivery, when performed by appropriately trained individuals, is safe and eliminates the significant risks associated with caesarean section when the fetal head is very low in the maternal pelvis.

KEY POINTS

- Induction of labour is offered to women with a low risk pregnancy at 41–42 weeks' gestation
- A membrane sweep should be offered to women at term to increase their chances of labouring spontaneously
- Bishop's score is generally used to determine the 'ripeness' or 'favorability' of the cervix, with scores of 6 or less suggesting an unfavourable cervix
- With an unfavourable cervix, induction of labour with vaginal prostaglandins is indicated
- Labour can be augmented when there is slow progress with an artificial rupture of membranes +/– oxytocin infusion. The frequency of uterine contractions and the fetal heart should be carefully monitored while on the oxytocin infusion

- Transcutaneous electrical nerve stimulation (TENS), Entonox, morphine and an epidural are all options for pain relief in labour
- Prior to performing an instrumental delivery, care must be taken to ascertain the position and station of the head vaginally, and to confirm that no more than one-fifth of the head is palpable abdominally. Where the head is in a position other than occipito-anterior (e.g. occipito-posterior or transverse), rotation to the occipito-anterior position can be performed either manually, with a ventouse or by rotational forceps and delivery completed

Further reading

NICE Clinical Guideline. *Intrapartum care: management and delivery of care to women in labour.* CG55, September 2007.

PART 2: CASES

Case 15 A 37-year-old woman with heavy bleeding per vaginum following a forceps delivery

Mrs Brown, a 37-year-old para 5, delivered by rotational forceps, was noted to have steady heavy bleeding per vaginum while in the recovery, 1 hour 30 minutes after delivery. You have been called to assess her.

What differential diagnosis would you be considering as a cause for postpartum haemorrhage (PPH)?

- Uterine atony
- Traumatic cause – vaginal or cervical tear
- Retained placenta or placental tissue
- Disseminated intravascular coagulation
- Uterine rupture
- Uterine inversion

KEY POINT

Primary postpartum haemorrhage (PPH) is defined as loss of more than 500 mL blood from the genital tract within 24 hours of delivery. Secondary PPH is vaginal bleeding of more than 500 mL after 24 hours and up to 6 weeks after delivery. Massive PPH is blood loss of more than 1.5 L.

What specific questions would you ask?

- What has the total blood loss since delivery been?
- What oxytocics have been administered so far?
- What are her pulse and blood pressure (BP) recordings?

Mrs Brown had lost about 400 mL blood vaginally while in recovery, with a steady trickle continuing. The total blood loss since delivery is estimated to be 850 mL. Her pulse rate is 96 beats/minute and her BP is 121/78 mmHg. She had syntometrine in the third stage of labour.

Obstetrics and Gynaecology: Clinical Cases Uncovered.
By M. Cruickshank and A. Shetty. Published 2009 by Blackwell Publishing. ISBN 978-1-4051-8671-1.

KEY POINT

Active management of the third stage of labour reduces the risk of atonic PPH. Ergometrine 500 μg with 5 units oxytocin is given by intramuscular injection immediately after the baby is delivered. Alternatively, 10 units oxytocin alone may be given by intramuscular injection if ergometrine is inappropriate as in cases of pre-eclampsia or cardiac disease.

What other relevant information would you wish to obtain?

- Was the placenta complete?
- What was the weight of the baby?
- Had labour been prolonged?

Mrs Brown has had five spontaneous vaginal deliveries in the past. There had been no complications in the previous pregnancies and deliveries.

In the current pregnancy there had been no problems antenatally, labour was induced at 40 weeks +12 days. Labour was augmented with oxytocin because of slow progress in the first stage and a rotational forceps delivery was performed in theatre for a prolonged second stage and occipito-transverse fetal position. The baby weighed 4.17 kg. Placenta and membranes were delivered completely and the episiotomy was sutured in layers. The total blood loss at the end of the procedure was 450 mL.

What features would you look for in your examination?

- Signs of pallor, pulse and BP
- On abdominal examination – level of the uterus in relation to umbilicus, tone of uterus (atonic or contracted)
- Assessment of the vaginal bleeding

Mrs Brown appears comfortable. There is no obvious pallor, her pulse is 96 beats/minute and her BP 121/78 mmHg. The uterus is palpable till the umbilicus and does not appear to be well contracted. A vaginal pad is fully soaked with blood and there is a persistent trickle continuing (Table 15.1).

What would be your initial management?

• IV access – two large (14 G) cannulae should be inserted
• Blood for full blood count (FBC), urea and electrolytes (U&E), coagulation screen, group and save and ask for at least 2 units of cross-matched blood
• Volume replacement with crystalloids followed by colloids
• Nasal oxygen 8–10 L/minute
• Catheterize the bladder
• Massage the uterus and perform bimanual compression (Fig. 15.1)
• Involve the senior obstetrician, anaesthetist and senior midwife at an early stage

A bolus of 500 μg ergometrine should be administered IV. A total of 1 mg ergometrine can be given if there is continued atony.

Give 5–10 units oxytocin as an IV bolus and oxytocin infusion (40 units oxytocin in 500 mL normal saline at a rate of 125 mL/hour) should be commenced IV.

> **Box 15.1 Predisposing factors for postpartum haemorrhage**
>
> • Uterine overdistention – multiple pregnancy, polyhydramnios, big baby
> • Prolonged labour
> • Antepartum haemorrhage – placenta previa, abruption
> • Grand multiparity (parity >5)
> • General anaesthesia

If the uterus remains atonic with persistent bleeding despite the above measures, 250 μg carboprost IM could be administered and repeated after 15 minutes, depending on the response to a maximum dose of 2 mg (eight doses).

Following administration of ergometrine, give an oxytocin bolus and oxytocin infusion.

Mrs Brown's uterus is well contracted, but there is still continued vaginal bleeding. The placenta appears complete. By now she has lost 1.6 L blood. Her pulse is 112 beats/minute, her BP is 96/50 mmHg and she appears pale. Her haemoglobin is 96 g/L and the coagulation profile is normal.

What is the next line of management?

• Head-down tilt
• Oxygen 8–10 L/minute by mask
• Hartman solution 2 L IV, Gelofusine 1.5 L IV
• Cross-match 6 units, O-negative blood if cross-match not ready

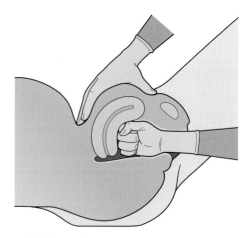

Figure 15.1 Bimanual compression.

Table 15.1 Clinical findings in obstetric haemorrhage.

Blood volume loss	Blood pressure (systolic)	Symptoms and signs	Degree of shock
500–1000 mL (10–15%)	Normal	Palpitations, tachycardia, dizziness	Compensated
1000–1500 mL (15–25%)	Slight fall (80–100 mmHg)	Weakness, tachycardia, sweating	Mild
1500–2000 mL (25–35%)	Moderate fall (70–80 mmHg)	Restlessness, pallor, oliguria	Moderate
2000–3000 mL (35–50%)	Marked fall (50–70 mmHg)	Collapse, air hunger, anuria	Severe

After ACOG educational bulletin. Hemorrhagic shock. *Int J Gynaecol Obstet* (1997) 57: 219–226.

- Communicate with the senior midwife, senior obstetrician, anaesthetist, haematologist, blood transfusion service and porter
- Continuous pulse/BP/oximeter
- Examination under anaesthesia (EUA) in theatre to rule out cervical, vaginal laceration and retained placental remnants (Boxes 15.2 & 15.3)

Mrs Brown has an EUA under general anaesthetic which shows bleeding from a cervical and vaginal tear. The uterus is contracted and found to be empty. A central venous pressure line is inserted by the anaesthetist. Cervical and *vaginal tears are sutured and haemostasis secured. Total blood loss by the end of EUA is 3.2 L. She receives 4 units blood and 1 unit of fresh frosen plasma. Prophylactic intravenous augmentin is administered (Figs 15.2 and 15.3; Box 15.4).*

What would be your postoperative management?

- Monitoring of pulse, BP, respiratory rate, oxygen saturation and temperature every 15 minutes
- Monitoring of hourly urine output
- Watch for vaginal bleeding
- Thromboembolic disease stockings and dalteparin if platelets and clotting are normal
- Repeat FBC, clotting profile and U&E

Box 15.2 Management of retained placental tissue

If the placenta has not been delivered before the onset of PPH, an attempt should be made to deliver it with cord traction and uterine countertraction. Care must be taken because the risk of uterine inversion is greater if the uterus remains poorly contracted. Manual removal should be performed under anaesthesia if the placenta is not easily delivered or the cord is avulsed.

If the placenta has been previously delivered, then exploration of the uterus is indicated if the uterus continues to relax when bimanual compression and massage are stopped despite the administration of uterotonics.

Inverted uterus

The uterus is said to be inverted if it turns inside-out during delivery of the placenta. Repositioning the uterus should be performed immediately.

Box 15.3 Management of genital tract trauma

Genital tract trauma is the most likely cause if bleeding persists despite a well-contracted uterus. EUA with suturing of vaginal or cervical laceration using absorbable suture material is indicated.

Lower genital tract haematomas are usually managed by incision and drainage, although expectant management is acceptable if the lesion is not enlarging. Any bleeding vessels are tied off, and oozing areas may be oversewn.

Broad ligament and retroperitoneal haematomas can be initially managed expectantly if the patient is stable and the lesions are not expanding. Ultrasound, CT scanning and MRI can all be used to assess the size and progress of these haematomas. Selective arterial embolization may be the treatment of choice if intervention is required in these patients.

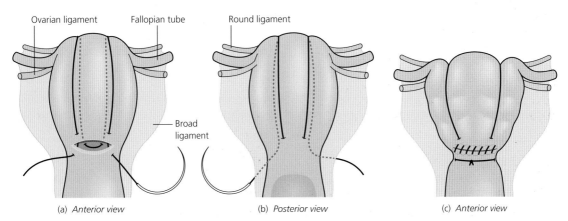

Figure 15.2 Insertion of the B-Lynch suture. (a) and (b) demonstrate the anterior and posterior views of the uterus showing the application of the B-Lynch Brace suture; (c) shows the anatomical appearance after competent application.

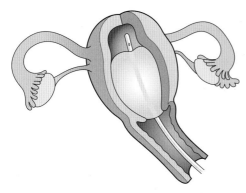

Figure 15.3 Bakri intrauterine balloon.

Box 15.4 Management of coagulopathy

If manual exploration has excluded genital tract trauma or retained placental fragments, bleeding from a well-contracted uterus is most commonly caused by a defect in haemostasis. Coagulation screen results clarify this diagnosis. Replacement with blood products is indicated. Cryoprecipitate may be useful along with fresh frozen plasma because of the markedly depressed fibrinogen levels. Cryoprecipitate provides a more concentrated form of fibrinogen and other clotting factors (VIII, XIII, von Willebrand factor).

Mrs Brown recovers very well. Her observations are stable with good urine output and minimal lochia. The repeat haemoglobin is 88 g/L, platelets 187 × 10⁻⁹/L, with normal U&E and clotting. She receives dalteparin until she is fully mobile and is started on 200 mg ferrous sulphate twice daily. She goes home on the fourth post-delivery day with follow-up arranged with the community midwife. The puerperium is uncomplicated until day 12 when she begins to feel unwell with some lower abdominal pain and increased lochia. The bleeding becomes heavier the following day and is also associated with a fever which brings her into the hospital.

What is the diagnosis and what do you think are the possible causes of the problem?

The diagnosis is secondary PPH. The two most common causes of secondary PPH are retained products of conception and intrauterine infection (endometritis).

What are the important features on history and examination?

A review of the hospital notes and delivery records to confirm completeness of the placenta, etc. Signs of pallor, pulse, temperature and BP should be checked.

On abdominal examination, the level of the uterus in relation to the umbilicus, signs of peritonism and uterine tenderness should be looked for. The vaginal loss should be assessed and a speculum examination carried out to see if the cervical os is open.

Mrs Brown's pulse is 88 beats/minute, BP 100/70 mmHg, temperature 38.1 °C, her abdomen is soft and she has moderate vaginal loss. The uterus was well involuted, tender and the cervix closed.

What is the most likely cause for PPH here and what investigations would you perform?

The diagnosis is endometritis as the uterus is involuted but tender and the cervix is closed and therefore retained placental remnants are unlikely in this case.

Blood should be taken for FBC, clotting profile, U&E, C-reactive protein, group and save, and 2 units of blood at least cross-matched.

An endocervical swab, high vaginal swab and blood cultures should also be taken.

What are the most likely organisms responsible for secondary PPH and what antibiotics would you administer?

The most likely organisms are anaerobes including bacteroids and peptostreptococci and the enteropharyngeal group which includes *Escherichia coli* and streptococci.

Antibiotics (intravenous while she remains pyrexial) may need to include metronidazole to cover anaerobes, aminoglycoside for Gram-negative organisms and cefuroxime to cover Gram-positive organisms.

Mrs Brown's haemoglobin level is 88 g/L, her white cell count 19.2 × 10⁹/L, platelets 332 × 10⁹/L, CRP 253 mg/L, and U&E and clotting are normal. The high vaginal swab grows Streptococcus viridans sensitive to augmentin. She responds well to antibiotics, her bleeding settles and she makes a good recovery.

Box 15.5 Surgical methods of managing atonic postpartum haemorrhage

If there is continued bleeding despite aggressive medical management, surgical management should be considered early.

Conservative measures
- *Packing of uterus:* packing the uterus with sterile gauze could be attempted, with the end of the pack fed through the cervix into the vagina
- *Balloon tamponade:* 'Bakri SOS' balloon, Sengstaken–Blakemore oesophageal catheter and the Rusch urological hydrostatic balloon are options for tamponade. The balloon is inflated with 100–300 mL warm 0.9% sodium chloride until enough counter-pressure is exerted to stop bleeding from uterine sinuses. The balloon tamponade is left in place for 6–8 hours to allow time for blood transfusion and coagulopathy correction. Once vital parameters are within acceptable limits, the balloon is deflated in two stages – half the 0.9% sodium chloride is withdrawn, and if there is no significant bleeding after

30 minutes, the remaining volume is withdrawn to deflate and remove the balloon.

Laparotomy
- *B-Lynch suture:* this involves opening the lower segment and passing a suture through the posterior uterine wall and then over the fundus to be tied anteriorly.
- *Uterine artery ligation*
- *Internal iliac artery ligation*
- *Hysterectomy:* this is curative for bleeding arising from the uterus or cervix While subtotal hysterectomy may be performed faster and be effective for bleeding caused by uterine atony, it may not be effective for controlling bleeding from the lower segment, cervix or vaginal fornices.

Uterine artery embolization
Interventional radiology should be considered in the management of PPH when surgical options have been exhausted, in managing haematomas, and with continued bleeding following hysterectomy.

CASE REVIEW

Mrs Brown was a grand multipara which increased her risk of atonic PPH and had a rotational forceps delivery which also put her at a higher risk of traumatic PPH. She received supportive care to maintain her circulating blood volume and oxygenation and treatment with oxytocics (ergometrine and oxytocin) which controlled the uterine atonicity. However, as the bleeding continued she had an EUA in theatre, both to see if there were tears of the cervix, vagina or uterus causing the continuing bleed and also to confirm an empty uterus without any retained remnants of placenta. The EUA revealed cervical and vaginal tears that were repaired and haemostasis achieved.

She presented some days later with a secondary PPH which was clinically and on investigation likely to be caused by an endometritis. This responded well to antibiotics. In view of her grand multiparity, Mrs Brown is at a higher risk of PPH in subsequent pregnancies.

Obstetric haemorrhage remains a problem both in terms of maternal mortality and severe morbidity. The incidence of severe bleeding in childbirth is estimated to be 5 per 1000 maternities. Dealing with an ill bleeding woman requires skilled teamwork between obstetric and anaesthetic teams with appropriate help from other specialists including haematologists, vascular surgeons and radiologists. Senior staff should be involved as early as possible.

Maternal tachycardia, severe abdominal pain and tenderness are important early features of genital tract sepsis. High-dose broad-spectrum intravenous antibiotics should be started immediately sepsis is suspected, without waiting for microbiology results. Disseminated intravascular coagulation and uterine atony are common in genital tract sepsis and often cause life-threatening PPH.

KEY POINTS

- Primary PPH can be caused by uterine atony, trauma to the genital tract, problems with coagulation or a combination of these. Secondary PPH may be brought about by endometritis and/or retained placental remnants
- With a significant PPH, resuscitation of the mother, supportive care, good communication with other specialities including anaesthetics and haematologists, and appropriate investigation and intensive monitoring is vital
- With a uterine atony, completeness of the placenta must be confirmed and measures instituted including administration of oxytocics and bimanual massage of the uterus

- When bleeding continues despite aggressive medical management, surgical management should be considered early. An EUA to rule out retained placental remnants or trauma of the genital tract should be undertaken in the first instance with recourse to other measures including ballon tamponade of the uterus, laparotomy and B-Lynch suture, as required
- With secondary PPH, management includes appropriate resuscitation, antibiotic treatment and evacuation of the uterus, if indicated

A 16-year-old woman with high blood pressure at 32 weeks gestation

Miss Jones is a 16-year-old primigravida who is 32 weeks' pregnant. At a routine antenatal check with her midwife her blood pressure is found to be 160/100 mmHg (mean arterial pressure [MAP] 120 mmHg).

Her midwife sends her to the maternity day assessment unit for review.

What differential diagnosis should you consider?
- Essential hypertension
- Secondary hypertension
- Pregnancy-induced hypertension
- Pre-eclampsia (Box 16.1).

What information do you need from the history?
• Does she have any symptoms that may be related to high blood pressure? Specifically, headache, visual disturbance, epigastric pain, nausea and vomiting.
• Does she have lots of swelling? Do her rings still fit? Does she feel her face is swollen?
• Is the baby moving? Has there been any abdominal pain or vaginal bleeding?
• Has she had any problems with the pregnancy to this point?
• What was her blood pressure at her booking appointment?
• Does she have any significant past medical history, especially renal disease or diabetes?
• Have any of her close family members had high blood pressure in their pregnancies?

Miss Jones tells you she is feeling absolutely fine, although she has had to take off her engagement ring and her fiancé

Obstetrics and Gynaecology: Clinical Cases Uncovered.
By M. Cruickshank and A. Shetty. Published 2009 by Blackwell Publishing. ISBN 978-1-4051-8671-1.

says her face looks puffy. She has been very well in the pregnancy to this point. There has been no bleeding or abdominal pain and baby is moving well.

She has no past medical history or family history of note. She cannot remember her booking blood pressure but you can see from her notes it was 100/60 mmHg.

What are the risk factors for pre-eclampsia
• First pregnancy, or first pregnancy with new partner
• Multiparous with:
  ◦ pre-eclampsia in any previous pregnancy
  ◦ 10 years or more since last baby
• Pregnancy at extremes of maternal age
• Body mass index (BMI) of 35 or more
• Family history of pre-eclampsia (in mother or sister)
• Booking diastolic blood pressure of 80 mmHg or more
• Booking proteinuria (of one or more, on more than one occasion or quantified at 0.3 g/24 hours or greater)
• Multiple pregnancy
• Certain underlying medical conditions:
  ◦ pre-existing hypertension
  ◦ pre-existing renal disease
  ◦ pre-existing diabetes
  ◦ antiphospholipid antibodies

What features will you look for on examination?
General examination
• Is she obviously oedematous? Remember 50% of pregnant women will have some peripheral oedema
• What are her pulse and blood pressure now?

Neurological examination
• Does she have normal upper and lower limb reflexes?
• Is there clonus? More than two beats is significant
• On fundoscopy, is there any evidence of papilloedema?

Box 16.1 Definitions

Pre-existing hypertension: defined as a systolic blood pressure of ≥140 mmHg, and/or a diastolic blood pressure of ≥90 mmHg, either pre-pregnancy or at booking (before 20 weeks)

Pregnancy-induced hypertension: develops after 20 weeks' gestation. May reflect a familial disposition to chronic hypertension or be an early manifestation of pre-eclampsia

Pre-eclampsia: pregnancy-induced hypertension in association with proteinuria ≥0.3 g in 24 hours with or without oedema

---

Box 16.2 Mean arterial pressure

- The average pressure within an artery over a complete cycle of one heartbeat:

$$MAP = 1/3 \text{ systolic pressure} + 2/3 \text{ diastolic pressure}$$

- An MAP of at least 60 mmHg is necessary to perfuse coronary arteries, brain, kidneys, etc.
- Usual range of MAP is 70–110 mmHg

Abdominal examination

On abdominal palpation:
- Is there tenderness in the right hypochondrium (over the liver)?
- Does the baby seem well grown?
- Lie and presentation of the baby
- Doppler fetal heart check

Which initial investigation do you request?

Urinalysis for protein.

Miss Jones looks well. Her BMI is 36 and she has moderate pitting oedema of her lower legs to mid calf. Her pulse is 86 beats/minute and her mean blood pressure over three readings using an appropriate-sized BP cuff is 155/95 mmHg (MAP 115; Box 16.2). She has normal reflexes and fundoscopy and no clonus. The baby seems a little small for gestational age with a symphysiofundal height of 29 cm. It has a longitudinal lie and cephalic presentation, the fetal heart is heard clearly. Her urinalysis shows ++ protein.

What is the most likely diagnosis based on the history and examination?

Pre-eclampsia.

Box 16.3 Blood tests in pre-eclampsia

Pre-eclampsia can affect any organ system but some investigations are especially helpful in suggesting an end organ effect

Urate
An increase in serum urate levels is often considered the 'early warning' blood test in pre-eclampsia and can indicate renal impairment before U&E becomes deranged

Urea and electrolytes
Indicates renal impairment. Note normal ranges for urea and creatinine are lower in pregnancy – get reference ranges from local laboratory

Liver function tests
Become abnormal in variants of pre-eclampsia with liver involvement especially in HELLP syndrome (haemolytic anaemia, elevated liver enzymes and low platelet count)

Full blood count
Can indicate HELLP with drop in haemoglobin secondary to haemolysis and low platelet count

Coagulation screen
Not routinely required but should be included in severe pre-eclampsia and if platelets are found to be abnormal

---

What would you do next?
- Admit her to the antenatal ward
- Carry out 4-hourly BP monitoring
- Fluid intake–output balance chart
- 24-hour urine collection for quantification of proteinuria
- Check full blood count (FBC), serum urea and electrolytes (U&E), liver function tests and urate (Box 16.3)
- Arrange an ultrasound scan for fetal size and well-being (Box 16.4; Figs 16.1 & 16.2)
- Administer corticosteroids for fetal lung maturity in case of worsening condition and need for delivery before 36 weeks (Box 16.5)

Miss Jones consistently has blood pressures below 160/100 mmHg so no treatment is required. Her urine output is good and all blood tests are normal. Ultrasound confirms that the baby is just above the 5th centile and has normal liquor volume. A first dose of steroids is given.

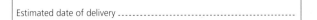

Estimated date of delivery --

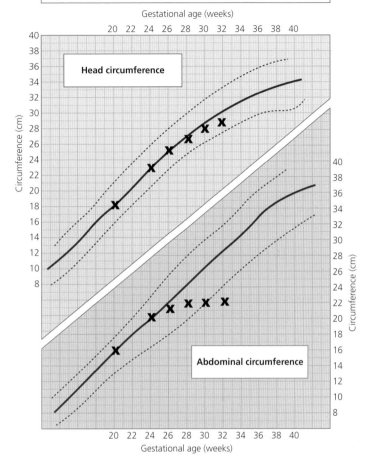

Gestational age (weeks)

Head circumference

Circumference (cm)

Abdominal circumference

Circumference (cm)

Gestational age (weeks)

Figure 16.1 Example of fetal growth chart.

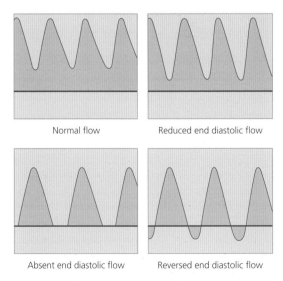

Normal flow

Reduced end diastolic flow

Absent end diastolic flow

Reversed end diastolic flow

Figure 16.2 Umbilical artery Doppler waveforms.

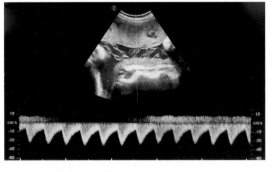

Figure 16.3 Normal umbilical artery Doppler.

Box 16.4 Intrauterine growth restriction

In pre-eclampsia, a combination of abnormal placentation and hypertension can result in reduced placental blood flow and fetal nutrition leading to intrauterine growth restriction (IUGR). IUGR is a term used to describe a baby that is smaller than expected for gestation; the usual cut-off is <5th centile for gestation. In addition to pre-eclampsia there are a variety of other problems that can result in IUGR.

Maternal factors
- High blood pressure
- Chronic kidney disease
- Advanced diabetes
- Heart or respiratory disease
- Malnutrition, anaemia
- Infection
- Substance abuse (alcohol, drugs)
- Cigarette smoking

Factors involving the uterus and placenta
- Decreased blood flow in the uterus and placenta
- Placental abruption (placenta detaches from the uterus)
- Placenta previa (placenta attaches low in the uterus)
- Infection in the tissues around the fetus

Factors related to the developing fetus
- Multiple gestation (twins, triplets, etc.)
- Infection
- Birth defects
- Chromosomal abnormality

It is important to identify these fetuses as babies with IUGR are at an increased risk of problems at birth including:
- Hypoxia/hypoxaemia
- Low Apgar scores
- Meconium aspiration
- Hypoglycaemia
- Hypothermia
- Polycythaemia

In addition, severe IUGR may result in stillbirth. It may also lead to long-term growth problems in babies and children.

If a fetus is found to be <5th centile for gestation, further ultrasound assessment including liquor volume, umbilical artery Doppler studies (umbilical arterial blood flow becomes abnormal when there is placental insufficiency) and biophysical profiles can help to distinguish those babies who are small but coping, from those babies who are struggling and will benefit from early delivery despite being premature (Figs 16.2 and 16.3).

Box 16.5 Drug choices for high blood pressure

It remains unclear whether antihypertensive drug therapy for mild to moderate hypertension during pregnancy is worthwhile. Antihypertensive treatment should be started in women with a systolic blood pressure >160 mmHg or a diastolic blood pressure >110 mmHg; MAP 125 mmHg.

In women with other markers of potentially severe disease, treatment can be considered at lower degrees of hypertension.

Labetalol (orally or intravenously), oral nifedipine or intravenous hydralazine can be used for the acute management of severe hypertension. Both labetolol and hydralazine can be given as IV boluses with or with out infusions.

ACE inhibitors, angiotensin receptor-blockers and diuretics should be avoided.

What will you tell Miss Jones about her condition?

She has a condition called pre-eclampsia. This is a combination of high blood pressure and protein in the urine. It is important because it can affect both the mother's and the baby's health. About 25% of women will get high blood pressure in their first pregnancy and 5/1000 women will develop severe pre-eclampsia. The only 'cure' for the condition is delivery of the baby and placenta.

However, as the baby is preterm and she is feeling well, as long as her blood pressure is satisfactory, all her blood tests are normal and baby is coping well (normal scans and cardiotocography [CTG]) the plan is to wait and monitor her and the baby until it is mature (≥37 weeks).

At 02.00 the next night Miss Jones calls the midwife to say she has a mild headache and could she have some paracetamol. The midwife checks her blood pressure and finds it to be 170/110 mmHg (MAP 130). She calls the doctor.

What will you do?

Attend as soon as possible. One per cent of women with severe pre-eclampsia will develop an eclamptic seizure which has a mortality rate of 1.8%, with 35% suffering severe morbidity.

Site IV access, check bloods as above plus urgent group and save and coagulation screen in case delivery is necessary.

Inform your senior and arrange transfer as soon as possible to a high dependency area (usually the labour ward).

Miss Jones' headache is now severe with a pain score of 9/10. She has no visual disturbance or epigastric pain but is hyper-reflexic and has marked clonus. Her blood pressure remains 170/110 mmHg (MAP 130) and she now has ++++ protein in her urine.

Box 16.6 Seizure prophylaxis

Magnesium sulphate should be considered when there is concern about the risk of eclampsia. In women with less severe disease, the decision is less clear and will depend on the individual case.

Magnesium sulphate is the therapy of choice to control seizures. A loading dose of 4g is given by infusion pump over 5–10 minutes, followed by a further infusion of 1g/hour maintained for 24 hours after the last seizure.

Recurrent seizures should be treated with either a further bolus of 2g magnesium sulphate or an increase in the infusion rate to 1.5g or 2.0g/hour.

During administration it can cause flushing and palpitations and cause the woman to feel quite unwell so it is important to warn her about this before commencing the treatment.

Box 16.7 Fluid balance

Fluid restriction is advisable to reduce the risk of fluid overload in the intrapartum and postpartum periods. Total fluids should usually be limited to 80 mL/hour or 1 ml/kg/hour.

Urine volumes of ≥0.5 mL/kg/hour are desirable. Usually, 30 mL/hour is acceptable.

Oliguria is common initially but if persistent its management should involve senior anaesthetic and obstetric staff and invasive monitoring of central venous pressure because of a significant risk of fluid overload and problems with pulmonary and cerebral oedema.

What are your priorities?

- Reduce her blood pressure
- Seizure prophylaxis (Box 16.6)
- Recheck blood pressure, re-examine and site catheter for urinalysis and hourly urine volumes
- Maintain strict fluid balance restricted to 80 mL/hour (Box 16.7)

Once the mother is stabilized perform CTG and arrange urgent delivery (Box 16.8).

KEY POINT

Magnesium toxicity is important as it can ultimately cause respiratory and cardiac depression and death. One of the earliest signs of toxicity is loss of deep tendon reflexes, and patellar tendon reflexes (or bicep tendon in the case of a woman with epidural or spinal anaesthetic) should be performed hourly during treatment.

Respiratory rate should also be monitored and, as magnesium is excreted in urine, if hourly urine volumes fall considerably it is sensible to halve the rate of infusion. Magnesium levels are not routinely monitored but if there was any clinical concern regarding toxicity stopping the infusion and taking a serum level may help with decision-making.

The antidote is calcium gluconate and this should be used immediately in cases of respiratory or cardiac depression.

Box 16.8 Choice of mode of delivery

The decision to deliver should be made once the woman is stable and with appropriate senior personnel present.

If the fetus is less than 34 weeks' gestation and delivery can be deferred, corticosteroids should be given, although after 24 hours the benefits of conservative management should be reassessed. Conservative management at very early gestations may improve the perinatal outcome but must be carefully balanced with maternal well-being.

The mode of delivery should be determined after considering the presentation of the fetus and the fetal condition, together with the likelihood of success of induction of labour after assessment of the cervix.

The third stage should be managed with 5 units Syntocinon IM or slow IV. Ergometrine and Syntometrine should not be given for prevention of haemorrhage, as this can further increase the blood pressure.

Miss Jones' blood pressure improves following 5 mg hydralazine IV to 145/90 mmHg. Her headache resolves with this treatment. She is commenced on magnesium sulphate for seizure prophylaxis. The CTG is satisfactory. Her cervix is unfavourable for induction of labour (Bishop score 3; see Case 1) and as her platelets and coagulation are normal a decision is made for emergency caesarean section.

An uncomplicated section is performed and a healthy male baby is delivered. As 44% of eclamptic seizures occur postnatally it is vital to remain vigilant so Miss Jones is transferred back to the high dependency unit.

What will be your plan for postnatal care?

Intensive monitoring of pulse, blood pressure and oxygen saturation every 15 minutes initially, reducing to hourly once she is completely stable. Also take hourly urine volume measurements. Administer magnesium sulphate for 24 hours following delivery and take hourly reflexes while she is on magnesium sulphate. Repeat blood tests at least daily until she is well. Use thromboembolic disease (TED) stockings and low molecular weight heparin for deep venous thrombosis prophylaxis if coagulation and/or platelet count is normal.

Miss Jones improves significantly over her first 24 hours postnatally. Her blood pressure remains stable and daily blood tests are normal. She is observed for a further 4 days on the postnatal ward before discharge. On day 2 her blood pressure is noted to be slightly elevated, she is commenced on oral antihypertensive therapy and her blood pressure improves. Her baby is doing well in the neonatal unit. She asks the midwife if she will always need tablets for her blood pressure now and if she will develop pre-eclampsia in her next pregnancy. The midwife calls you to talk to her before discharge.

What will you tell her?

Most women who develop pre-eclampsia become completely better over a period of days to weeks but some women will require treatment for longer. Her GP will check her blood pressure regularly and stop her tablets when she no longer needs them. If her blood pressure is high at 6 weeks they will refer her for investigation of this.

More women who have pre-eclampsia will develop high blood pressure in later life compared with the whole female population. Women who have pre-eclampsia in a first pregnancy are at an increased risk (7–10%) of developing it in a subsequent pregnancy.

Miss Jones is happy with your explanation and is discharged to the care of her GP. An appointment for a postnatal check is made with her consultant for 6 weeks' time in view of her severe pre-eclampsia.

CASE REVIEW

Miss Jones, in view of her age of 16 years and being in her first pregnancy, had risk factors for developing pre-eclampsia. As in most cases, pre-eclampsia was first picked up on routine antenatal screening with BP and urine protein checks which are performed at every antenatal visit. She demonstrated some of the complications of pre-eclampsia including a small baby and signs of impending eclampsia with a significant increase in her blood pressure. Prophylaxis for eclampsia was with magnesium sulphate and the blood pressure was controlled rapidly with hydralazine IV. The only treatment for pre-eclampsia is delivery of the baby and once maternal condition was stabilized delivery was planned. As her cervix was unfavourable with a low Bishop's score, an emergency caesarean section was performed. Her monitoring continued postpartum as the risks of severe pre-eclampsia remain for some time postnatally.

Pre-eclampsia is a common and serious complication of pregnancy. There are specific factors that put women at increased risk of pre-eclampsia but it can occur in anyone. Severe pre-eclampsia can affect any maternal organ system and can cause fetal intrauterine growth restriction (IUGR) and placental abruption.

Five in 1000 women will develop severe pre-eclampsia and 5 in 10,000 will have an eclamptic seizure. Of these, 38% of seizures occur antenatally, 18% intrapartum and 44% postnatally.

Low dose aspirin prophylaxis may be beneficial in preventing recurrence of pre-eclampsia when there has been early onset of severe disease with or without IUGR.

Appropriate management of blood pressure can sometimes prolong pregnancy but the only cure for pre-eclampsia is delivery of baby and sometimes this will have to be at an early gestation despite the risks to the fetus.

KEY POINTS

- Extremes of maternal age, first pregnancy (or first pregnancy with a new partner) and multiple pregnancy are some of the risk factors for pre-eclampsia
- Maternal complications of pre-eclampsia include HELLP, renal failure, disseminated intravascular coagulopathy, pulmonary odema, intracerebral haemorrhage and eclampsia. Over 40% of eclamptic fits occur postpartum
- Fetal complications include IUGR, increased perinatal and neonatal morbidity and mortality, mostly due to IUGR and prematurity (which is very likely to be iatrogenic)
- Headaches, visual disturbances, epigastric and/or right hypochondrial tenderness and hyper-reflexia suggest worsening of pre-eclampsia and/or impending eclampsia.

Magnesium sulphate is the treatment of choice for eclampsia and prophylaxis of eclampsia
- Antihypertensives are indicated with MAP readings of 125 or above (or with systolic readings ≥160 mmHg and diastole ≥110 mmHg)
- Close monitoring of blood pressure, fluid intake and output, and blood investigations (including haemoglobin and platelet counts, U&E, liver function tests) is indicated with severe pre-eclampsia
- In the presence of oliguria, central venous pressure monitoring should be considered before fluid challenges to avoid the risks of fluid overload and pulmonary and cerebral odema

Further reading

The management of severe pre-eclampsia/eclampsia. RCOG Green topped Guideline No 10 (A), March 2006.

Case 17   A 34-year-old woman with painless vaginal bleeding at 33 weeks' gestation

Mrs Chou, a 34-year-old woman in her third pregnancy, presents to the maternity day assessment unit with a history of bleeding per vaginum (PV) about an hour prior to presentation. She is 33 weeks' pregnant.

What differential diagnoses would you consider as a cause for the antepartum haemorrhage?

- Placenta praevia
- Placental abruption
- Local (cervical, vaginal) causes
- Preterm labour
- Bleeding of uncertain origin

KEY POINT

Antepartum haemorrhage (APH) is defined as bleeding from the genital tract after about 24 weeks' gestation and is seen in 3–5% of pregnancies. About half of cases turn out to be bleeding of unknown origin after the other causes listed above are ruled out with appropriate investigation and examination.

What specific questions would you wish to ask about her presenting symptoms?

- Has there been any abdominal pain?
- How much has she bled? Has it been fresh bleeding? Any clots? Any fluid leaking PV?
- Has she been feeling the baby move?
- Is this the first episode of bleeding?
- Did she have sexual intercourse prior to the bleed?

Mrs Chou says that there has been no pain. This was the first episode of bleeding. The bleeding has been fresh, but a

small amount, about two teaspoonfuls. She has been feeling the baby move well, and there has been no change in fetal movements from previously. There is no history of intercourse over the last week.

What other relevant information would you wish to obtain?

- Obstetric details of her last two pregnancies:
  - gestation at delivery (term or preterm)
  - mode of delivery (vaginal or caesarean section)
  - any complications (e.g. APH, premature rupture of membranes)
- Has she been up to date with her cervical smears?
- What is her blood group?

Mrs Chou's first delivery was 4 years ago when she had an elective caesarean section at 39 weeks for the indication of a breech presentation. There had been no other antenatal complications, and her daughter weighed 3250 g at birth.

Her last pregnancy had been 2 years ago when she had an emergency caesarean section at 41 weeks for the indication of slow progress in labour. There had been no particular problems antenatally and she had gone into labour spontaneously. Her son weighed 3500 g at birth and was well. She had made a good postoperative recovery after both caesarean sections.

Mrs Chou was up to date with her cervical smears and had her last smear a year ago. All her smears to date have been negative.

Her blood group is O-negative. She received anti-D immunoglobulin antenatally and postnatally in both her previous pregnancies. She was administered prophylactic anti-D in this pregnancy at 28 weeks' gestation.

What features would you look for in your examination?

- Does she look distressed or in pain?
- Any signs of pallor, pulse and blood pressure recordings

Obstetrics and Gynaecology: Clinical Cases Uncovered.
By M. Cruickshank and A. Shetty. Published 2009 by Blackwell Publishing. ISBN 978-1-4051-8671-1.

- On abdominal palpation:
  - any tenderness
  - uterine tone and contractions
- Lie and presentation of the baby
- Doppler fetal heart check
- Check pads or undergarments stained with blood that the patient may have brought in, or for any signs of bleeding down her legs.

Mrs Chou appears comfortable. There is no obvious pallor, her pulse is 86 beats/minute and BP 130/76 mmHg. There is no tenderness on abdominal palpation, and the uterus is soft with no contractions. The baby is in the transverse position. The fetal heart is regular at around 140 beats/ minute. She is wearing a pad stained with a small amount of fresh blood.

What would be your most likely differential diagnoses based on the history and examination?
Placenta praevia.

> **KEY POINT**
>
> Placenta praevia must be considered in pateints with painless APH. Other pointers or risk factors to consider in the diagnosis of placenta praevia:
> - Previous caesarean section (especially multiple caesarean sections)
> - Fetal malpresentation or abnormal lie in the third trimester
> - Previous history of placenta praevia
> - Multiple pregnancy
> - Increasing age and parity
> - Placenta noted to be lying over the internal os at routine mid-trimester fetal anomaly scan

What would you do next?
- Fetal cardiotocography (CTG) to check fetal well-being
- Arrange an ultrasound scan for placental localization
- Kleihauer test and anti-D immunoglobulin as required
- *Avoid vaginal examination.*

The CTG is reassuring. The scan suggests a major anterior placenta praevia (grade III – placenta just extending over the cervical internal os; Box 17.1; Figs 17.1 & 17.2).

> **Box 17.1 Grades of placenta praevia as diagnosed on ultrasound**
>
> | | |
> |---|---|
> | Grade I | The placenta encroaches into the lower uterine segment (within 5 cm of the internal os) |
> | Grade II | The lower edge of the placenta reaches but does not cover the internal os |
> | Grade III | The placenta covers the internal os partially |
> | Grade IV | The placenta is centrally located over the internal os |
>
> Grade I and II are classified as 'minor' and grades III and IV as 'major' placenta praevia. The incidence of morbidity and mortality in the fetus and mother increases as the grade increases.

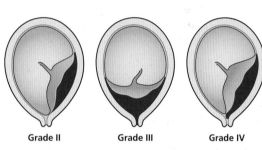

Figure 17.1 Grades of placenta praevia.

> **!RED FLAG**
>
> Avoid vaginal examination until the scan confirms that the placenta is not low lying. If placenta praevia is confirmed, avoid vaginal examination as it may trigger a torrential vaginal bleed.

Pain associated with APH should alert the clinician to a placental abruption or preterm labour (see Cases 18 and 19). In about 10% of women, placental abruption can occur with a low lying placenta and the two conditions can be present together.

If placenta praevia is ruled out on the scan, a speculum examination to visualize the cervix to look for lesions on the cervix (e.g. ectropin, polyp or, rarely, a malignancy) should be performed.

When the placenta is situated on the posterior wall of the uterus, transabdominal sonography may not be able to establish the grade of praevia adequately, especially if the patient is obese or the bladder is overdistended.

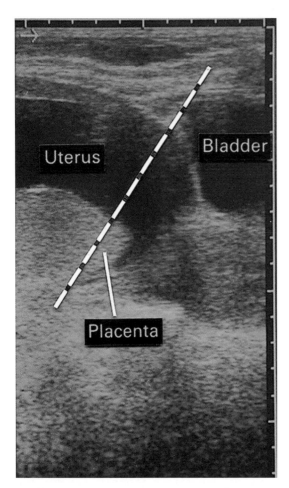

Figure 17.2 Posterior placenta praevia on transvaginal scan.

Transvaginal sonography may be required in these cases. There is no evidence that a gentle transvaginal scan triggers a vaginal bleed.

When placenta praevia is diagnosed with a history of previous caesarean section, an attempt must be made to look for scan features of placenta accreta or percreta. This includes indentifying a clear plane between the uterine wall and the placental bed. MRI imaging may also facilitate the diagnosis.

What features would you consider in making a management plan?
• Is there any further bleeding and if so, is it heavy?
• Are there any features of maternal or fetal compromise?
• What is the gestation?

There is no further bleeding. The mother's vital signs remain stable and fetal CTG remains reassuring.

What would be your management plan now?
Carry out expectant management until fetal maturity. Then plan for elective caesarean section at around 37–38 weeks if the placenta remains low lying.

Consider steroids for fetal lung maturity in case the bleeding becomes heavy, with fetal or maternal compromise, and delivery has to be considered before 36 weeks. Carry out serial scans every 2–4 weeks to check if praevia resolves as the uterus grows and lower segment increases. Group and save sample available at blood transfusion service at all times (preferably cross-matched blood if available). Discuss blood transfusion with the patient in the event of heavy bleeding. Give haematinics to maintain a normal haemoglobin.

Mrs Chou has two further small APHs and she remains in hospital. Scans at 35 and 37 weeks confirm that the placenta remains low grade III anterior. Her elective caesarean section is planned for 38 weeks' gestation. Scans do not suggest a placenta accrete or percreta.

Vaginal delivery may be considered in women where the placental edge is ≥2cm from the internal os and the fetal head is below the placenta edge as seen on the scan.

RCOG guidelines (2005) advise that women with major placenta praevia who have bled should be admitted and managed as inpatients. 'Those with major praevia who remain asymptomatic, require careful counselling before contemplating outpatient care. Any home based care requires close proximity with the hospital (can get into hospital within about 20minutes), the constant presence of a companion and full informed consent from the women.'

Even with minor praevia, if there are repeated episodes of PV bleeding, inpatient care may be recommended.

What might you discuss with her regarding the caesarean section?
There is an increased risk of bleeding at caesarean section for placenta praevia. Blood transfusion should be rediscussed. In view of the two previous caesarean scars and the placenta being situated anteriorly and over the old scars, there remains the risk of the placenta being

adherent, although the scans do not confirm this. An adherent placenta increases the risk and amount of postpartum haemorrhage (PPH) and if this is not controlled by conservative measures, a hysterectomy may be required to control the bleeding.

Regional anaesthesia may lower the blood pressure, which may worsen things if there is active bleeding, so a general anaesthetic is the usual anaesthetic of choice when bleeding is anticipated.

KEY POINT

Postpartum haemorrhage may occur after the separation of a low lying placenta, owing to the inability of the lower segment to contract efficiently and arrest bleeding from vascular sinuses.

Previous reports on the Confidential Enquiries into Maternal Deaths have recommended that a senior anaesthetist and obstetrician must be available at the caesarean section. Cross-matched blood must also be available.

Mrs Chou has her lower segment caesarean section performed electively at 38 weeks' gestation. The placenta is encountered on making the uterine incision and is sheared away from the uterine wall to get to the baby. The baby is delivered feet first as it is still in the transverse position. The placenta is removed complete. There is increased bleeding from the lower segment placental bed. An oxytocin bolus is administered soon after delivery of the baby and an infusion of oxytocin is ongoing to facilitate uterine contraction. Some of the larger vascular areas on the lower segment are controlled with haemostatic sutures. The bleeding is brought under control, and the operation completed satisfactorily. Blood loss at surgery is 2000 mL.

Her haemoglobin checked on day 1 postoperatively is 9.8 g/dL (preoperative level was 12.1 g/L) She is given dalteparin prophylaxis until fully mobile on day 5 postoperatively for the prevention of thrombosis (risk factors for thrombosis include the pregnancy, surgery, increased blood loss and prolonged hospitalization which might have resulted in reduced mobility). She is also continued on her haematinics with advice to continue these until her haemoglobin is rechecked 4–6 weeks later and confirmed as normal.

CASE REVIEW

Mrs Chou developed a major placenta praevia diagnosed on scan at 33 weeks' gestation when she presented with painless bleeding PV and a fetal malposition (transverse lie). Her two previous caesarean sections increased her risk of having a low lying placenta. She was managed conservatively until fetal maturity. In view of repeated APHs she was managed as an inpatient.

Repeat scans showed the placenta to remain as a major praevia and an elective caesarean section was planned for 38 weeks. In view of her risks of PPH at caesarean section, a senior obstetrician and anaesthetist were present at her surgery with cross-matched blood available. While she did have a blood loss of 2000 mL, the surgery proceeded without event and she made a good postoperative recovery.

In view of this being her third caesarean section, future deliveries would be advised through an elective caesarean section. She would also be counselled about the increased risks of both a low lying and an adherent placenta and of an uncontrolled PPH that might necessitate a hysterectomy.

When the blastocyst implants low in the uterine cavity, placenta praevia may occur. Scarring of the uterine cavity (e.g. from previous caesarean section) or a large placenta (e.g. with multiple pregnancy) predispose to a placenta that lies in the lower uterine segment.

While around 25% of placentae are seen to be low lying at the second trimester scan, this reduces to 5% at 32 weeks and <0.5% at term with increasing development of the lower segment. The recurrence of placenta praevia is approximately 2%.

There is usually some bleeding in the third trimester to suggest a low lying placenta, along with a fetal malpresentation in one-third of women. However, in fewer than 2%, bleeding is seen only in labour.

Antepartum or postpartum haemorrhage is the main cause of maternal morbidity, and premature delivery the main cause of fetal problems. Most of the episodes of APH settle spontaneously and conservative treatment to attain fetal maturity beyond 36 weeks may be attempted to the extent of blood transfusions for the heavier bleeds, with careful observation of mother and fetus.

KEY POINTS

- Placenta praevia must be considered in those with painless vaginal bleeding
- Risk factors for or associations with placenta praevia include previous caesarean section (especially multiple caesarean sections) and malpositions of the fetus
- Vaginal examinations must not be performed where there is a suspicion of placenta praevia until an ultrasound scan has ruled it out
- A transvaginal scan may provide clearer views of the placenta in the lower segment (especially with a posterior placenta) than a transabdominal scan

- If the bleeding settles and there is no maternal or fetal compromise, expectant management until fetal maturity is advised
- With grade II, III and IV placenta praevia, elective caesarean section around 38 weeks is the preferred mode of delivery. Vaginal delivery may be considered if the lower edge of the placenta is 2 cm or more from the internal cervical os, with the fetal head below the placental edge
- There is the risk of PPH with a low lying placenta as the lower segment does not contract as effectively as the upper segment after separation of the placenta

---

Further reading

Bhide A, Prefumo F, Moore J, Hollis B, Thilaganathan B. Placental edge to internal os distance in the late 3rd trimester and mode of delivery in placenta praevia. *Br J Obstet Gynaecol* 2003; 110: 860–864.

Royal College of Obstetricians and Gynaecologists Guideline (Green Top) no 27. *Placenta praevia and placenta praevia accrete: diagnosis and management.* RCOG Press, London, October 2005.

Case 18   A 39-year-old woman with painful vaginal bleeding at 37 weeks' gestation

Mrs O'Neil, a 39-year-old woman, is brought into the labour ward by ambulance at 37 weeks' gestation in her fourth pregnancy. She gives a short history of sudden onset worsening abdominal pain and bleeding per vaginum.

What differential diagnoses would you consider?
- Placental abruption
- Placenta praevia (see Case 17)
- Early labour
- Other causes (e.g. cervical or vaginal polyps, cervical ectopy)
- Unexplained

What history would you like to elicit from this patient to help you formulate a diagnosis?
Presenting complaints
- Nature and site of pain – is it constant or intermittent?
- Amount and nature of bleeding – is it fresh and with clots, exclude 'show' mixed with liquor?
- Fetal movements – are they present?
- History of problems in present pregnancy (e.g. pre-eclampsia)

Past obstetric history
Details of previous pregnancies and labours including complications such as placental abruption, placenta praevia or intrauterine growth restriction.

Past medical, personal and social history
- Cervical smear history
- History of hypertension
- Smoking or cocaine use

Obstetrics and Gynaecology: Clinical Cases Uncovered.
By M. Cruickshank and A. Shetty. Published 2009 by Blackwell
Publishing. ISBN 978-1-4051-8671-1.

Mrs O'Neil had been feeling somewhat off colour for the past day or so, although prior to that her pregnancy had been uneventful. Earlier today she experienced worsening abdominal pain along with a small amount of dark red vaginal bleeding. She feels this pain is different from her previous labours as it was constant and did not feel like uterine contractions. She had not felt her baby move since the pain set in.

She has had three uneventful pregnancies all resulting in vaginal deliveries at term. In her present pregnancy, she booked at 18 weeks and has seen her midwife on two occasions as documented in her handheld notes. She smokes 25–30 cigarettes every day but denies substance abuse and lives in a council house with her three children.

What key signs would you look for during the physical examination?
General examination
Check for pallor. Take her pulse and blood pressure.

Abdominal examination
Check the symphysiofundal height, fetal lie and presentation. If uterine contractions are present, what is their strength, duration and frequency. Is the uterus relaxing well between contractions?

Check for tenderness on abdominal palpation. What is the tone of the uterus between contractions (i.e. is it soft, or hypertonic/hard/woody)?

Assess the fetal heart rate.

Mrs O'Neil is pale and in obvious pain. Her pulse is 132 beats/minute and her BP is 90/60 mmHg. The uterine height is appropriate for gestation, although it is difficult to ascertain the fetal lie as her uterus feels woody hard and is tender to touch. The midwife is unable to pick up the fetal heart on Doppler ultrasound or cardiotocography (CTG). There is minimal dark red blood loss per vaginum.

Now let us reconsider the diagnosis on the basis of the information available

Mrs O'Neil's history and clinical examination are highly suggestive of mixed type placental abruption leading to

---

Box 18.1 Placental abruption

This occurs in approximately 1 in 80 deliveries

Definition
The partial or complete premature separation of the placenta prior to the birth of the baby

Risk factors
• Increasing maternal age and/or parity
• Low socioeconomic group
• Smoking or cocaine use
• Hypertensive disorders
• Sudden uterine decompression (e.g. rupture of membranes with polyhydramnios)
• Severe external trauma
• Uterine abnormality, short cord
• Previous history of abruption. Recurrence rate is 7–9%

Symptoms
• Abdominal pain – usually constant and severe with backache
• Vaginal bleeding – may be old or fresh blood
• Reduced or absent fetal movements

Signs
• Shock out of proportion to blood loss
• Spasm of uterus – described as 'woody' – from hypertonic contractions
• Tender uterus
• Fetal parts difficult to feel
• Often no fetal heart
• Rarely may present as idiopathic preterm labour

Classification
• *Concealed:* blood trapped between the placenta and uterine wall, no external bleeding
• *Revealed:* blood tracks between the membranes and uterine wall with external bleeding from placenta edge separation
• *Mixed:* combination of both types

---

shock and intrauterine fetal death as the cause for her antepartum haemorrhage (APH) (Boxes 18.1 & 18.2; Fig 18.1). The other common cause of APH, placenta praevia, is usually associated with a painless APH in which the shock is in proportion to the external bleeding. Also, as the bleeding is maternal, the fetus is usually in good condition. This is therefore an unlikely diagnosis in Mrs Smith's case.

What are the complications associated with placental abruption?

Placental abruption is a condition frequently associated with serious maternal morbidity and high perinatal morbidity and mortality (Box 18.3).

What would be the next step in the management of the mother?
Resuscitation of the mother

• Call for help from the senior obstetrician, anaesthetist and midwifery staff
• Check airway, breathing and circulation (ABC) and give oxygen. Insert two large-bore intravenous cannulae and start fluid resuscitation by crystalloid or colloid (Box 18.4)
• Determine the patient's rhesus status and cross-match blood (4–6 units)
• Alert porters, laboratories and the blood bank
• Obtain blood for a full blood count, biochemistry (urea and electrolytes, serum creatinine and urate, liver function tests) and coagulation screen

---

Box 18.2 Pathophysiology of placental abruption

• Placental abruption arises from haemorrhage into the decidua basalis of the placenta
• Expanding haematoma leads to separation of adjacent placenta with or without vaginal bleeding and fetal distress or demise
• Bleeding may be concealed wholly or in part
• Bleeding into the amniotic sac leads to bloodstained liquor
• Bleeding may infiltrate into the myometrium, tracking to the serosa and resulting in the appearance of a Couvelaire uterus
• Sustained uterine contraction is thought to be the result of intramyometrial bleeding and the release of prostaglandins

---

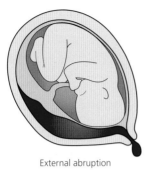 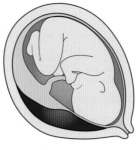 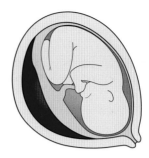

External abruption   Relatively concealed abruption   Concealed abruption

Figure 18.1 Concealed, revealed and mixed types of placental abruption.

Box 18.3 Complications of placental abruption

- Hypovolaemic shock
- Disseminated intravascular coagulation
- Postpartum haemorrhage
- Renal failure

Fetal complications
- Fetal distress
- Intrauterine fetal death
- Preterm delivery
- Perinatal mortality: 300/1000

Box 18.4 General management principles of obstetric emergencies

- Manage airway, breathing and circulation
- Remember, there are *two* patients – the mother and the fetus (although in this case there has been intrauterine fetal death)
- The fetus is vulnerable to maternal hypoxia

• Consider invasive monitoring (e.g. central or arterial line)
• Insert a urinary catheter for monitoring output and check for proteinuria
• Replace blood and blood products as required

Assess fetal health

Assess by ultrasound and CTG if the fetus is alive. Check fetal heart and lie and begin continuous fetal CTG. Also, look for the presence of retroplacental clot, which is not always evident on the scan, and confirm that the placenta is not low lying.

Delivery of the fetus

If the fetus is alive, the decision regarding the mode of delivery depends upon presence or absence of fetal distress, and the amount of haemorrhage. A caesarean section may be indicated for fetal or maternal reasons (e.g. deterioration of maternal condition, fetal distress as confirmed by CTG). If the fetus is not distressed, induction or augmentation of labour with artificial rupture of membranes with or without oxytocin infusion may be attempted with the aim of a vaginal delivery; however, the fetal condition must be closely and continuously monitored by CTG. If the fetus is dead, induction of labour may be performed if maternal condition allows.

Women with severe abruption usually labour spontaneously and tend to have short labours.

KEY POINT

Treatment is aimed at treating the shock and preventing disseminated intravascular coagulopathy (DIC).

Mrs O'Neil is managed as an obstetric emergency in the high dependency area of the labour ward. Immediate help is summoned and resuscitation commenced by giving facial oxygen and inserting two 14-gauge cannulae for fluid administration. Blood samples are obtained for urgent cross-match and relevant investigations and a urinary catheter inserted for output monitoring.

Intrauterine fetal death is confirmed by an onsite scan. The scan also confirmed partial separation of an anteriorly placed placenta by a large retroplacental clot.

A vaginal examination is performed which reveals that Mrs O'Neil is in labour and her cervix is 4 cm dilated. An amniotomy (artificial rupture of membranes) is performed and an infusion of Syntocinon commenced to expedite delivery. Liquor is noted to be bloodstained, consistent with the diagnosis of placental abruption.

Mrs O'Neil's condition remains stable over the next 20 minutes and the uterine contractions become more regular. Soon thereafter she delivers a fresh stillborn fetus weighing 3320 g. The placental delivery was followed by the passage of 950 g of old clots, confirming the diagnosis of placental abruption.

What would you watch out for after delivery?

Abruption increases the risk of atonicity of the uterus and postpartum haemorrhage (PPH). PPH can worsen or cause DIC.

Following the completion of the third stage of labour, the emergency buzzer is set off, as there is significant atonic PPH. Help is summoned and the haemorrhage is controlled by bimanual uterine compression and the administration of oxytocics. While the resuscitation is being carried out the anaesthetist notices that there is excessive oozing from the venepuncture sites along with significant bruising of her arm along the blood pressure cuff site, and haematuria. He suspects that DIC has set in and alerts the resuscitation team to the possibility. The on-call haematologist confirms the diagnosis of DIC.

The International Society on Thrombosis and Haemostasis defines DIC as: 'An acquired syndrome characterized by the intravascular activation of coagulation with loss of localization arising from different causes.'

With placental abruption, decidual fragments containing activated coagulation factors enter the maternal circulation. DIC in abruption is caused by enhanced and sustained abnormal generation of thrombin by intrinsic pathways of coagulation.

What are the diagnostic tests for DIC?

DIC is primarily a clinical diagnosis; laboratory tests are used to confirm the diagnosis and monitor replacement of blood components. No one test can diagnose DIC.

Tests for DIC
- Platelet count ↓
- Prothrombin time ↑
- Thrombin time usually ↑
- Activated partial thromboplastin time ↑
- Fibrinogen ↓
- Fibrinogen degradation products
- Microangiopathic changes on peripheral smear

How will you manage Mrs O'Neil, who has now developed DIC secondary to placental abruption?

- Continue to manage ABC
- Mainstay of management is to treat the underlying cause (e.g. if still undelivered, expedite delivery)
- Manage in consultation with a haematologist
- Laboratory tests dictate the need for blood, fresh frozen plasma, clotting factors replacement and platelet transfusion

Mrs O'Neil is managed by a multidisciplinary team comprising a consultant obstetrician, consultant anaesthetist and consultant haematologist along with supporting staff in a high dependency setting. Fluid replacement is guided by invasive monitoring, urine output and infusion of Syntocinon is used to maintain uterine contractility.

Packed red cells, fresh frozen plasma and cryoprecipitate are administered and over the next few hours her clinical condition stabilizes and her coagulation profile improves. She is monitored intensively for 24 hours with frequent relevant investigations.

She is then transferred to a single room in the postnatal ward caring for women with pregnancy loss. The following day a debriefing session is undertaken to go through the events and answer any questions. She is discharged home on day 4 following delivery, with a date for postnatal follow-up at the counselling clinic 6 weeks post delivery.

CASE REVIEW

This 39-year-old parous woman presented at 37 weeks' gestation in shock with a history of painful APH and loss of fetal movements. Her age, parity, smoking history and socioeconomic status place her at risk for placental abruption. Her history of constant abdominal pain, vaginal bleeding and the findings of a tender woody uterus along with fetal demise are highly suggestive of the diagnosis of placental abruption.

The mainstay of management is adequate resuscitation of the mother. The guidelines for managing major obstetric haemorrhage recommend that two peripheral lines should be set up using at least 14-gauge cannulae and blood cross-matched for 6 units. Plasma expansion should be provided by colloids.

The next step is to expedite delivery of the fetus, the mode of which depends upon gestation, fetal well-being and maternal condition. If the mother's condition is stable and the fetus is in good condition, induction of labour is appropriate, as women with abruption usually have a quick short labour.

Following delivery, PPH and DIC are the major complications to watch out for.

KEY POINTS

- Placental abruption is an important cause of maternal morbidity and perinatal morbidity and mortality
- Differential diagnosis is mainly from placenta praevia and labour
- APH with sustained painful uterine contractions in the presence of a tender uterus and fetal distress or demise should alert one to the diagnosis
- Multidisciplinary team involvement is strongly recommended
- Resuscitation of the mother and early delivery of the fetus are the mainstay of management
- PPH and DIC are serious complications to watch out for

Further reading
Baskett TF, Arulkumaran S. Antepartum haemorrhage. *Intrapartum Care for the MRCOG and Beyond*. RCOG Press. 2002; 133–141.

Hl-adky K, Yankowitz J, Hansen WF. Placental abruption. *Obset Gynecol Surv* 2002; 57: 299–305.

Case 19 A 29-year-old woman with leaking fluid per vaginum at 31 weeks' gestation

Ms McRoberts, a 29-year-old para 3 + 0, presented to the labour ward at 31 weeks' gestation with a history of a gush of fluid per vaginum in the early hours of the morning. She had been on her way to the toilet when she noticed fluid running down her legs. She had undergone a routine check with her midwife 2 days ago, when she was told that all was well with the pregnancy.

What would be the differential diagnosis here?
- Preterm premature rupture of membranes (PPROM)
- Urinary incontinence
- Vaginal discharge

KEY POINT

PPROM is defined as prelabour rupture of membranes prior to 37 completed weeks of gestation. It complicates 2% of pregnancies but is associated with 40% of preterm deliveries.

What specific information would you need from her history to help you formulate a diagnosis?
Presenting complaints
- Colour and amount of the fluid
- Any associated abdominal pain/contractions?
- Has she felt the baby move?
- Any urinary symptoms (e.g. dysuria and frequency)?
- Any flu-like symptoms?
- Any problems in the present pregnancy?

Past obstetric history
Details of her previous pregnancies and labours:
- Gestation at delivery (term or preterm)
- History of PPROM
- Spontaneous or induced labour
- Mode of delivery (vaginal or by caesarean section)
- Any complications

Past medical history including allergies
Is there anything of relevance in her past medical history and does she have any allegies?

Ms McRoberts has had an uneventful pregnancy until tonight. She denies any abdominal pain or contractions and reports normal fetal movements. She experienced a sudden gush of clear fluid on her way to the toilet. The fluid ran down her legs and wet the bathroom floor. She gives no history of dysuria but reports increased urinary frequency for the past week or two. Apart from that she had been feeling well and denies any major medical problems or allergies. She admits to smoking up to 20 cigarettes per day.

She has had three previous pregnancies. In her first two pregnancies she laboured spontaneously and had uneventful vaginal deliveries at term, while in the third pregnancy she had a preterm vaginal birth at 33 weeks' gestation following PPROM and then preterm labour. She gives no history of postnatal problems.

What key features would you look for on physical examination?
General examination
Signs of labour – does she appear to be in pain? Check her pulse, blood pressure and temperature recordings: tachycardia and pyrexia may indicate an infection.

Abdominal examination
- Uterine contractions
- Lie and presentation of the baby and symphysiofundal height

Obstetrics and Gynaecology: Clinical Cases Uncovered.
By M. Cruickshank and A. Shetty. Published 2009 by Blackwell Publishing. ISBN 978-1-4051-8671-1.

- Tenderness on palpation (sign of infection)
- Fetal heart check with Doppler and cardiotocograph (CTG)
- Pad check for colour of fluid

Ms McRoberts appears anxious but not in any pain. Her pulse is 90 beats/minute, her BP is 110/70 mmHg and her temperature is 36.8 °C. On palpation, the uterus is relaxed and non-tender with the fetus presenting as cephalic. The fundal height is appropriate to her gestation. The CTG appears reassuring with a normal reactive baseline of approximately 140 beats/minute, with accelerations.

What would you do next?
Speculum examination
The next step would be a sterile speculum examination looking for pooling of fluid in the posterior vaginal fornix to confirm spontaneous rupture of membranes. A convincing history followed by demonstration of presence of fluid in the posterior vaginal fornix is highly suggestive if not conclusive of rupture of membranes and further diagnostic tests are unnecessary. A high vaginal swab is obtained for culture and sensitivity at this time.

However, in case of equivocal findings it may be necessary to proceed to further diagnostic tests to confirm or refute the diagnosis of PPROM.

What additional diagnostic tests could you use?
1 *The nitrazine test.* A series of tests have been used to confirm membrane rupture; the most widely used has been the nitrazine test:
  ○ Detects pH change
  ○ Has a sensitivity of 90% and false positive rate of 17%
  ○ Normal vaginal pH is 4.5–6.0 (nitrazine paper does not change colour). With ruptured membranes, vaginal pH is 7.1–7.3 (colour of paper changes to blue)
  ○ A false positive test (nitrazine positive, pH >7) indicates blood, semen, antiseptic solutions or bacterial vaginosis

More recently, other tests (e.g. fetal fibronectin and raised insulin-like growth factor binding protein-1 in cervical or vaginal secretions) have reported sensitivities of 94% and 75%, and specificities of 97%, respectively.

2 *Ultrasound for liquor volume.* Ultrasound is useful in some cases to help confirm the diagnosis of PPROM, by demonstrating oligohydramnios (reduced liquor volume).

3 *Mid-stream sample of urine (MSSU).* MSSU should be obtained at this stage if other tests are negative to exclude a urinary tract infection.

A sterile speculum examination was performed which revealed obvious pools of clear fluid in the posterior vaginal fornix.

In view of the convincing history of rupture of membranes at 31 weeks' gestation and the presence of pools of liquor on speculum examination, the diagnosis was that of PPROM.

> **!RED FLAG**
>
> Digital examination should be avoided where PPROM is suspected.

> **Box 19.1 Preterm premature rupture of membranes**
>
> - PPROM leads to significant neonatal morbidity and mortality
> - The three causes of increased neonatal morbidity and mortality are prematurity, sepsis and pulmonary hypoplasia
> - Maternal risks are associated with chorioamnionitis
> - Women with intrauterine infection deliver earlier than non-infected women and infants born with sepsis have a mortality rate four times higher than those without sepsis
>
> **Risk factors associated with PPROM**
> - History of PPROM in previous pregnancy
> - Tobacco use
> - Amniocentesis or cervical cerclage in present pregnancy
> - History of cone biopsy of cervix
> - Uterine distension resulting from polyhydramnios and multiple pregnancy
> - Cervical or vaginal infection (e.g. bacterial vaginosis, group B streptococci, ureaplasma, *Chlamydia*)
>
> **Course prior to delivery**
> - *Term PROM:* labour starts within 24 hours in 70% of cases
> - *PPROM between 28 and 34 weeks:* labour starts within 24 hours in 50% of cases; labour starts within 1 week in 80% of cases
> - *PPROM between weeks 24 and 26:* labour starts within 1 week in >50%; labour delayed 4 weeks in 22%

Digital vaginal examination is best avoided unless there is a strong suspicion that the woman may be in labour. This is because microorganisms may be transported from the vagina into the cervix, leading to intrauterine infection, prostaglandin release and preterm labour.

What would be your plan of management?

1. *Assess fetal well-being.* Use fetal CTG and ultrasound to assess fetal well-being. Use ultrasound to establish the fetal growth and lie, and amniotic fluid volume.

2. *Exclude maternal infection* by:
- Regular observations – pulse, temperature, uterine activity and tenderness
- Blood tests – full blood count, C-reactive protein (CRP)
- High vaginal swab – chorioamnionitis is an ascending infection

---

KEY POINT

The criteria for the diagnosis of clinical chorioamnionitis include maternal pyrexia (>37.8°C), tachycardia, leucocytosis, uterine tenderness, offensive vaginal discharge and fetal tachycardia (>160 beats/minute).

During inpatient observation, the woman should be regularly examined for such signs of intrauterine infection as an abnormal parameter or a combination can indicate intrauterine infection (Box 19.2).

Box 19.2 Royal College of Obstetricians and Gynaecologists (RCOG) recommendations for monitoring for intrauterine infection

- Women should be observed for signs of clinical chorioamnionitis at least 12-hourly
- A weekly high vaginal swab and at least a weekly maternal full blood count should be considered
- Fetal monitoring using CTG should be considered where regular fetal surveillance is required
- Biophysical profile scoring or Doppler velocimetry should not be considered as first-line surveillance or diagnostic tests for fetal infection

---

The ultrasound scan shows that Ms McRoberts' baby is presenting as cephalic, is well grown and in good condition, with reduced amniotic fluid volume. She is apyrexial with a normal white cell count and has a CRP of <10. An high vaginal swab has been reported as negative.

What would you do next?
Prophylactic antibiotics

The use of antibiotics following PPROM was associated with a statistically significant reduction in chorioamnionitis. There was a significant reduction in the numbers of babies born within 48 hours and 7 days. Neonatal infection was significantly reduced in the babies whose mothers received antibiotics. Erythromycin (250 mg orally 6-hourly) should be given for 10 days following the diagnosis of PPROM. Co-amoxiclav is not recommended for women with PPROM because of concerns about necrotizing enterocolitis.

Corticosteroids

Antenatal corticosteroids should be administered in women with PPROM as steroids reduce the risks of respiratory distress syndrome, intraventricular haemorrhage and necrotizing enterocolitis. They do not appear to increase the risk of infection in either the mother or the fetus.

KEY POINT

Betamethasone is the steroid of choice to enhance lung maturation. Recommended therapy involves two doses of 12 mg betamethasone, given intramuscularly 24 hours apart.

The optimal treatment–delivery interval for administration of antenatal corticosteroids is more than 24 hours but fewer than 7 days after the start of treatment.

Ms McRoberts wonders whether she should receive drugs to prevent onset of labour to enable her to complete the course of corticosteroids.

Could tocolytic agents be used?

Evidence suggests that prophylactic tocolysis in women with PPROM without uterine activity is not recommended. The only indication for the short-term use of tocolytics could be to complete the course of steroids for fetal lung maturity or to allow for *in utero* transfer of the mother to a unit with neonatal facilities to manage a preterm neonate.

Ms McRoberts enquires about when she might be delivered?

Delivery should be considered at 34 weeks' gestation.

Where expectant management is considered beyond 34 weeks' gestation, women should be counselled about the increased risk of chorioamnionitis and its consequences versus the decreased risk of serious respiratory problems in the neonate, admission for neonatal intensive care and caesarean section. Therefore, it is standard practice to manage expectantly until 34 weeks' gestation.

Ms McRoberts is commenced on erythromycin as per protocol and also receives the first betamethasone injection. The neonatal unit is informed of her admission to ensure there is an available neonatal bed. The plan is for expectant management and induction of labour at 34 weeks' gestation. She feels well and wonders if she could be managed as an outpatient as she lives near the hospital and is willing to come for regular check ups and blood tests.

Can Ms McRoberts be managed as an outpatient?

In a randomized study of home versus hospital management outcomes, the two groups were comparable with a similar latency period and gestational age at delivery. There were no significant differences in the frequencies of chorioamnionitis, respiratory distress syndrome or neonatal sepsis (Box 19.3).

A management plan is made for Ms McRoberts to be monitored as an inpatient for 72 hours and then for discharge home, if all remains well. However, later that day she experiences abdominal discomfort and reports irregular uterine activity. Her observations are normal and the CTG is reassuring. On palpation she is noted to have one to two mild contractions every 15 minutes. The registrar on duty performs a sterile vaginal examination, which shows the cervix to be 1–2 cm dilated and shortened. The diagnosis is that of threatened preterm labour.

Ms McRoberts is extremely worried about her baby's health as she has not completed her steroid course and asks the registrar if anything could be done to stop her from labouring?

> **Box 19.3 RCOG recommendations for outpatient management in PPROM**
>
> - Women should be considered for outpatient monitoring of PPROM only after rigorous individual selection
> - Outpatient monitoring should be considered only after a period of 48–72 hours of inpatient observation
> - Women being monitored at home for PPROM should take their temperature twice daily and should be advised of the symptoms associated with chorioamnionitis (e.g. abdominal pain, pyrexia, change in the colour, smell of the fluid leaking per vaginum), and when they should seek specialist advice
> - There should be clearly described local arrangements for the frequency of outpatient visits and what should be carried out at these visits

> **Box 19.4 Tocolytic agents**
>
> A variety of preparations are available of comparative efficacy but different side-effect profiles
> - *Atosiban:* oxytocin antagonist
> - *Nifedipine:* calcium-channel antagonist
> - *Ritodrine (beta-agonist):* not preferred because of maternal side-effects
> - *Indometacin (antiprostaglandin):* concerns about safety in fetus and neonate
> - *Nitric oxide donors mainly glyceryl trinitrate:* under trial, comparative effectiveness to beta-agonist but fewer maternal side-effects
> - *Magnesium sulphate:* popular in the USA, comparative effectiveness to ritodrine but better tolerated

There is no clear evidence that tocolysis improves pregnancy outcome. Tocolysis should be considered if the few days gained would be put to good use, such as completing a course of corticosteroids or *in utero* transfer.

Once a decision is made to use a tocolytic drug, which is the best choice?

Atosiban or nifedipine appear preferable to ritodrine, a beta-agonist, as they have fewer adverse effects and seem to have comparable effectiveness (Box 19.4). Atosiban (an oxytocin antagonist) is licensed for tocolysis in the UK but nifedipine (a calcium-channel blocker) is not. Ritodrine has been the most thoroughly evaluated but, like all beta-agonists, has a high frequency of unpleasant and sometimes severe adverse effects (Box 19.5).

Box 19.5 Side-effects of tocolytic drugs

Maternal side-effects

Common: nausea, headache, dizziness, tachycardia, palpitations, chest pain

   Rare: hypotension, hyperglycemia, pulmonary oedema (beta-agonists)

   Atosiban is associated with fewer maternal side-effects than beta-agonists

Fetal side-effects

- Fetal and neonatal tachycardia
- Premature closure of ductus arteriosis, renal and cerebral vasoconstriction, necrotizing enterocolitis (indometacin)

After discussion, Ms McRoberts is commenced on the tocolytic drug atosiban and monitored in accordance with the departmental guideline in the high dependency area. Over the next few hours she feels more comfortable, her contractions settle and she manages some sleep overnight. Her observations remain stable on the infusion. She receives the second dose of betamethasone IM the following morning, and is transferred to the antenatal ward for observation after the ward round. The management plans remain as before: if she does not labour for outpatient management and induction of labour around 34 weeks' gestation.

   Ms McRoberts is discharged from hospital 72 hours later with follow-up planned at the day assessment unit, with advice regarding monitoring for the warning signs of chorioamnionitis. She starts to labour spontaneously 1 week later, comes into hospital and is delivered of a baby boy in good condition weighing 1956 g. The baby is transferred to neonatal unit in view of his prematurity. Her postnatal period is uneventful and she is discharged home 2 days later. Over the next few weeks her baby makes good progress in the neonatal unit requiring minimal ventilatory support and is discharged home 4 weeks later.

CASE REVIEW

Ms McRoberts presented with a convincing history of PPROM with no evidence of labour. She was a heavy smoker with a past obstetric history of preterm delivery and PPROM, thus putting her at a high risk of these recurring again in this pregnancy.

   The diagnosis was confirmed by a speculum examination. Normal recordings and relevant investigations confirmed maternal and fetal well-being. She was commenced on prophylactic antibiotics and prescribed steroids for fetal lung maturity, with a plan for conservative management until 34 weeks' gestation in the absence of chorioamniotis. However, before the course of steroids was complete she developed signs of labour. Tocolysis in the form of atosiban infusion was started to enable her to complete the course of steroids. Thereafter she was managed as an outpatient as the uterine contractions settled down and there was no evidence of chorioamnionitis.

   Premature labour set in within a week and she had a spontaneous vaginal delivery. Prior to discharge she was counselled about her increased risk of PPROM and preterm labour in subsequent pregnancies. This woman would be a candidate for detection and treatment of asymptomatic infections (e.g. bacterial vaginosis) by means of high vaginal swab in the second and early third trimesters along with prophylactic steroids (at around 28–29 weeks) for fetal lung maturity.

KEY POINTS

- Preterm labour is the single most important determinant of adverse infant outcome, most morbidity and mortality being experienced by babies born before 34 weeks
- *Definition:* onset of labour prior to 37 completed weeks of gestation
- *Incidence:* 6–15% of deliveries
- *Risk factors* for preterm labour include:
  - low socioeconomic status
  - extremes of maternal age
  - tobacco use or substance abuse
  - prior preterm delivery or second trimester miscarriage
  - African-American race
  - uterine anomaly (e.g. unicornuate or bicornuate uterus)
  - genitourinary infection
  - uterine distension caused by twins, polyhydramnios
  - history of cervical cone biopsy
- *Prediction of PTL:* various scoring systems exist, incorporating:
  - history of preterm delivery
  - assessment of cervical length: transvaginal ultrasound is the most sensitive test
  - fetal fibronectin: high negative predictive value
  - research tools: salivary oestriol, home monitoring
- *Prevention:*
  - prophylactic cervical cerclage if cervical incompetence is suspected
  - detection and treatment of asymptomatic infections in high risk women (e.g. bacterial vaginosis, asymptomatic bacteriuria)
- *Treatment:*
  - emergency cerclage/rescue cervical suture (limited evidence)
  - tocolysis: no clear evidence that it improves outcome. Should be considered if the few days gained would be put to good use, such as completing a course of corticosteroids or *in utero* transfer. Evidence suggests no benefit of antibiotic use in women with intact membranes.

Further reading

Royal College of Obstetricians and Gynaecologists. *Tocolytic drugs for women in preterm labour.* Green-top Guideline No.1 (B). RCOG, London, 2002.

Royal College of Obstetricians and Gynaecologists. *Antenatal corticosteroids to prevent respiratory distress syndrome.* Green-top Guideline No. 7. RCOG, London, 2004.

Royal College of Obstetricians and Gynaecologists. *Preterm prelabour rupture of membranes.* Green-top Guideline No. 44. RCOG, London, 2006.

A 35-year-old woman booking for antenatal care

Mrs Todd is a 35-year-old woman in her third pregnancy. Her last menstrual period (LMP) was 12 weeks ago and she has been well in this pregnancy up until now. She is attending for her first antenatal visit.

Antenatal screening is designed to identify those pregnancies at greater risk of complications. It comprises information from the history, as well as ultrasound scanning, blood tests and other investigations. As a result of cost and clinical effectiveness, only screening tests recommended by the National Institute for Health and Clinical Excellence (NICE) are included here, although other screening tests are indicated during some pregnancies.

What information do you need from the history?

1 Past obstetric history
   ○ Number and outcomes of previous pregnancies
   ○ Any problems with the pregnancies including:
      ○ pre-eclampsia, abruption, etc.
      ○ mode of delivery
      ○ gestation at delivery
      ○ birth weights
      ○ any postnatal problems
2 Past medical history
3 Drug history, including allergies
4 Social history
   ○ Ethnicity
   ○ Occupation
   ○ Social support
   ○ Smoking
   ○ Alcohol intake
   ○ Illicit drug use
5 Family history, including partner and his family

Obstetrics and Gynaecology: Clinical Cases Uncovered.
By M. Cruickshank and A. Shetty. Published 2009 by Blackwell Publishing. ISBN 978-1-4051-8671-1.

She tells you that her first two pregnancies were uncomplicated vaginal deliveries at term of normal-sized babies. She has no significant past medical history or allergies and does not take any medicines. She is a legal secretary, does not drink alcohol or use illicit drugs but smokes 30 cigarettes per day. She is adopted and unable to provide any information regarding family history but there are no problems on her husband's side.

What advice will you offer at this stage?

She should try to cut down or stop smoking. If her partner smokes they could stop together. Smoking cessation advice, support groups and nicotine replacement therapy are all available in pregnancy via referral from maternity services or her GP.

She accepts your offer to refer her for smoking cessation advice as she realizes it is detrimental to hers and her baby's health.

She has read the leaflet that the hospital sent about screening in pregnancy but is very unclear and would like you to explain it to her.

What would you discuss with her?

Screening in pregnancy is designed to detect conditions that have no symptoms but can have detrimental effects on her or her baby. They usually comprise blood tests, urine tests and ultrasound scanning. They aim to detect infections, fetal abnormalities and abnormalities in the maternal blood (Boxes 20.1 & 20.2). Screening is also available for some medical conditions that can affect the pregnancy.

Mrs Todd accepts haematological screening and screening for infection. She tells you she is very worried about the risk of Down's syndrome in this pregnancy as her neighbour had a baby with Down's syndrome after low risk screening. She asks you if she can have an ultrasound scan to make sure her baby does not have Down's syndrome.

Box 20.1 Screening for haematological conditions

Anaemia

Adequate haemoglobin concentrations prevent symptoms and reduce the need for postnatal blood transfusion. The most common cause of anaemia in pregnancy is iron deficiency. Screening for anaemia should be offered at booking and 28 weeks. This allows time for treatment if anaemia is detected.

Hb levels <11 g/dL at booking or <10.5 g/dL at 28 weeks should be investigated with a serum ferritin. Levels <30 μg/L indicate inadequate iron stores and supplementation should be prescribed.

Blood grouping and red cell alloantibodies

Identifying blood group, rhesus D status and red cell antibodies is important in preventing haemolytic disease of the newborn and to identify potential transfusion reactions. Identifying rhesus D-negative women also allows them to be offered appropriate antenatal and postnatal immunoprophylaxis to try to prevent rhesus D alloimmunization in subsequent pregnancies.

Current recommendations are testing of ABO, rhesus D typing and screening for irregular antibodies at booking and 28 weeks' gestation.

Sickle cell disorders and thalassaemia

Haemoglobin disorders are autosomal recessive but it is possible to inherit more than one. They can cause a variety of illnesses of varying severity and the aim of screening is to identify women at risk in early pregnancy so that genetic counselling can be provided and they can make a decision about invasive diagnostic tests and continuation of their pregnancy.

Screening can be based on a combination of an ethnicity question to identify women at higher risk, then investigation of the high risk group for haemoglobin abnormalities, or on offering laboratory screening to all pregnant women.

What will you tell her?

Ultrasound is a useful test for many fetal abnormalities but is not a good test for Down's syndrome as many babies with Down's syndrome appear normal on scan.

Screening tests are available for Down's syndrome and other chromosomal abnormalities but only provide a risk of the pregnancy being affected. That means that low risk results do not definitely mean the baby is unaffected (false negatives). Conversely, a high risk result does not definitely mean the baby is affected (false positives). The simplest test of risk is based on maternal age. At 20 years the risk is 1 in 1440 rising to 1 in 32 aged 45. Mrs Todd's age related risk at 35 years is 1 in 338. Other screening tests involve combinations of blood tests, ultrasound scans and some information from the mother's history.

If a screening test has a high-risk result (usually >1 in 250), because the baby is not definitely affected the parents would be offered a diagnostic test (amniocentesis or chorionic villous sampling [CVS]) to provide a definitive diagnosis.

Mrs Todd understands what you have told her and does not think she wants to have an amniocentesis straight away but would consider it if she was uncomfortable with the results of the screening tests. She asks you for more information about the available tests.

It is important to discuss with her the methods, timing and possible consequences of screening, including the possibility of being faced with a decision about termination of an affected pregnancy. You should also discuss the options available for screening in your hospital. Screening for Down's syndrome includes screening the pregnancy for some other chromosomal abnormalities (e.g. trisomy 13 and 18; Boxes 20.3 & 20.4; Fig. 20.1). You should tell her that she can change her mind and opt out of the screening programme at any time.

She is happy to accept the combined test and has her booking scan and NT performed. She has a 12-week singleton continuing pregnancy with neural tubes within the normal range. The midwife performs her booking bloods along with the pregnancy-associated plasma protein A (PAPP-A) and human chorionic gonadotrophin (hCG) as part of the combined test (Box 20.5).

At 20 weeks she returns to the hospital for her detailed ultrasound scan. The combined test gave the pregnancy a risk of Down's syndrome of 1 in 1775 and Mrs Todd and her partner are reassured by this. They wonder if they still need the detailed scan.

Box 20.2 Screening for infections

Asymptomatic bacteriuria

Persistent bacterial colonization of the urinary tract occurs in 2–5% of pregnant women in the UK. Pregnant women with asymptomatic bacteriuria have an increased risk of pyelonephritis and preterm birth. Treatment with antibiotics reduces these risks.

It is therefore recommended that all pregnant women be screened for this with mid-stream urine culture early in pregnancy and treated with appropriate antibiotics if it is detected.

Hepatitis B virus infection

Hepatitis B infection is often asymptomatic and may be highly infectious. Mother–child transmission results in a significant proportion of chronic carriage in the baby and chronic carriage results in a high risk of hepatocellular carcinoma and cirrhosis. Approximately 95% of mother–child transmission is preventable through the administration of vaccine and immunoglobulin to the baby at birth.

Therefore, all pregnant women should be offered serum screening for hepatitis B infection to allow effective postnatal intervention to be offered. Immunoglobulin administration and hepatits B vaccination for babies of infected women reduces the risk of mother–child transmission.

HIV

The prevalence of HIV in women of reproductive age is increasing in the UK. In the absence of intervention, mother–child transmission occurs in around 25% of deliveries. Appropriate interventions (see Case 26) can reduce this figure to <1%.

All pregnant women should be offered screening for HIV antibodies early in pregnancy so appropriate interventions can be put in place to reduce vertical transmission.

Rubella

Rubella infection in early pregnancy can have catastrophic consequences. There is no treatment to prevent or reduce mother–child transmission of rubella for the current pregnancy. Screening for rubella antibodies enables susceptible women to be vaccinated in the postnatal period for the protection of future pregnancies.

Syphilis

Syphilis is rare now in the indigenous UK population but may be more common in the increasing immigrant population.

In pregnant women with early untreated syphilis, 70–100% of babies will be infected and one-third will be stillborn. Mother–child transmission is associated with neonatal death, congenital syphilis (which may cause long-term disability), stillbirth and prematurity.

Early detection and parenteral treatment of the mother with penicillin effectively prevents mother–child transmission. The outcome of treated pregnancies with syphilis is comparable with the outcome of pregnancies in women who never had syphilis. Screening also allows for appropriate referral to genitourinary medicine (GUM) services and treatment of the mother. Therefore, despite the rarity of the condition as a result of the efficacy of available treatment and serious consequences of non-treatment, screening continues.

Box 20.3 Screening for Down's syndrome (trisomy 21) and other common chromosomal abnormalities

Antenatal screening can take place in the first or second trimester. It is recommended that the test performed should have a detection rate above 75% for a false positive rate less than 3% (NICE guideline on antenatal screening; see further reading). The tests all have advantages and disadvantages in terms of timing and false positive and negative rates but meet the above criteria as a minimum.

11–14 weeks – the combined test

Nuchal translucency (NT) measures the subcutaneous space between skin and cervical spine in early pregnancy. Increased measurements are associated with increased risk (Fig. 20.1). This measurement is used in combination with maternal serum levels of human chorionic gonadotrophin (hCG) and

pregnancy-associated plasma protein A (PAPP-A). The NT can usually be performed with the booking scan.

14–20 weeks – the quadruple test

Maternal serum is sent for the quadruple test that comprises hCG, alpha-fetoprotein (AFP), unconjugated estriol (uE3) and inhibin A.

11–14 weeks *and* 14–20 weeks

The integrated test – NT, PAPP-A + hCG, AFP, uE3, inhibin A
plus
the serum integrated test – PAPP-A + hCG, AFP, uE3, inhibin A

Box 20.4 Screening for neural tube defects

A maternal serum AFP carried out between 15 and 21 weeks can indicate a high risk for neural tube defects (NTDs). A value >2 mean of median is considered high risk and these women would be offered detailed ultrasound scans to look for a cause for the elevated AFP.

Problems other than NTDs that may cause an elevated AFP:

- Inaccurate pregnancy dating
- Bleeding in early pregnancy
- Multiple pregnancy
- Fetal death
- Abdominal wall defects – gastroschisis or exomphalos

Sometimes an elevated AFP is unexplained and these pregnancies remain at increased risk of intrauterine growth restriction, preterm delivery and pre-eclampsia, closer surveillance of these pregnancies may be warranted.

If routine detailed ultrasound scanning is offered to all women at 20 weeks' gestation, most of the abnormalities resulting in an elevated AFP would be detected and it may be unnecessary to offer this test in addition to a routine detailed ultrasound scan.

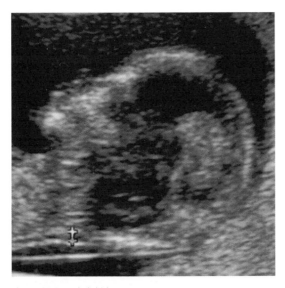

Figure 20.1 Nuchal thickness on scan.

Box 20.5 Diagnostic tests

If a pregnancy is found to be at high risk of a chromosomal abnormality the woman then has the option of an invasive diagnostic test to identify the karyotype of the fetus.

Chorionic villous sampling (CVS) can be performed between 10 and 14 weeks' gestation. It takes a tiny amount of tissue from the placenta and carries a 2% risk of miscarriage (Fig. 20.2).

Amniocentesis can be performed from 15 weeks' gestation. Amniotic fluid is withdrawn from around the fetus and the fetal fibroblasts in the fluid are cultured to give the fetal karyotype. It carries approximnately 1% risk of miscarriage (Fig. 20.3). The provisional result is usually available after 24–72 hours (from quantitative fluorescence polymerase chain reaction [QF-PCR]) with a full karyotype in a few weeks.

In addition to the risk of miscarriage, there is an approximtely 1% risk of mosaicism, culture failure and requiring repeat testing depending on which test is undertaken.

What would you discuss with her regarding the mid-trimester anomaly scan?

The screening test she has already had was for the common trisomies. The detailed ultrasound aims to detect structural abnormalities in the baby. However, detailed ultrasound scans do not detect all abnormalities. If any abnormalities are detected during this screening scan a more detailed scan will be offered. If the baby has a major abnormality it may mean having to reach a decision about whether or not to continue with the pregnancy. It can also give valuable information regarding a problem that may require specialist paediatric services, and may help with deciding the place of birth of a baby with a known abnormality (Box 20.6; Fig. 20.4; Table 20.1).

Mrs Todd is happy to have her detailed ultrasound scan which shows that her baby appears structurally normal. She is very reassured and able to relax through the latter half of her pregnancy.

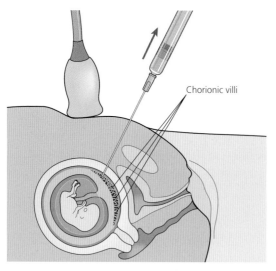

Figure 20.2 Chorionic villus sampling.

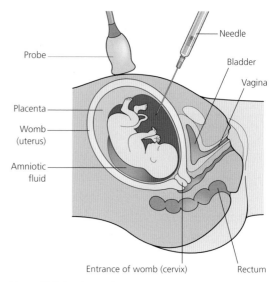

Figure 20.3 Amniocentesis.

Box 20.6 Detailed ultrasound scan

Many abnormalities can be detected on mid-trimester ultrasound:
- Cleft lip
- Ventricular and atrial septal defects
- Diaphragmatic herniae
- Absent or abnormal kidneys
- Gastroschisis and exomphalos (Fig. 20.4)
- Spina bifida
- Limb abnormalities

The detection rates vary with the:
- Type of abnormality being screened
- Gestational age at scanning
- Skill of the operator
- Quality of the equipment
- Time allotted for the scan

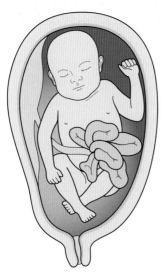

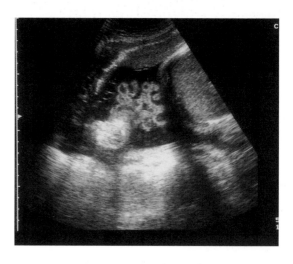

Figure 20.4 Gastroschisis.

Table 20.1 Percentage of fetal abnormalities detected by routine ultrasound screening in the second trimester (evidence level IIa). As detection rates vary, all departments providing detailed scanning services should monitor their own results and provide local detection rates to assist patient's decision-making about detailed ultrasound scan.

Anatomical system	Detected (%)
Central nervous system	76
Urinary tract	67
Pulmonary	50
Gastrointestinal	42
Skeletal	24
Cardiac	17

CASE REVIEW

Screening in pregnancy aims to detect asymptomatic conditions that may have a detrimental effect on the pregnancy. Usually, screening for haematological conditions and infections, is reasonably straightforward but adequate counselling is required in case of an unexpected positive result.

The issue of screening for fetal abnormality is particularly difficult. There are a number of problems regarding the woman's understanding of the concept of risk. In addition, there is the potential need for subsequent testing for the woman to grasp. It is important that she understands the implications of screening. The fact that a diagnosis of fetal abnormality may lead to a decision about termination of pregnancy needs to be handled sensitively before screening begins.

KEY POINTS

- All screening tests for fetal chromosomal aneuploides and abnormalities can have false positive and false negative results. It is important that a woman is fully informed about the implications of screening and of both a high and a low risk result
- Screening tests for Down's syndrome include those that can be performed in the first and/or the second trimester and include risk calculation based on combinations of maternal age + blood tests or age + NT scanning or age + blood tests + NT scanning
- When there is a high risk result on a screening test, a diagnostic test (CVS or amniocentesis) is indicated to confirm the fetal karyotype. Both of these procedures have a procedure-related fetal loss rate
- Routine antenatal screening for infections include that for hepatitis B, HIV and syphilis. In these infections, measures can be taken to reduce fetal effects of the maternal infection. With screening for rubella, when non-immunity is confirmed, rubella vaccination is indicated postnatally to protect future pregnancies
- Other screening tests may be indicated in high risk groups (e.g. screening for sickle cell in women of African origin or for thalassaemia in the Mediterranean populations)

Further reading

Antenatal care: routine care for the healthy pregnant woman.
  NICE Clinical Guideline CG62, March 2008.

Case 21 A 24-year-old insulin-dependent diabetic woman planning a pregnancy

Ms Kumar is a 24-year-old known to have type 1 insulin-dependent diabetes mellitus (IDDM) since the age of 15 years. She is in a stable relationship and wishes to start a family.

What prepregnancy advice and care would you offer her?

Offer prepregnancy counselling and care by a multidisciplinary team (combined obstetric and diabetic clinic) as good control of diabetes and lower HbA1c levels lower the risk of congenital malformations in the fetus and are associated with improved pregnancy outcome.

Review her medication and intensify her hypoglycaemic therapy to aim for HbA1c <6.1%.

Advise continuation or commencement of contraception until good glycaemic control is achieved (HbA1c <6.1%) as the risk of congenital malformations with levels >10% can be as high as 25%. Carry out monthly measurement of HbA1C and increase the frequency of self-monitoring of blood glucose. The aim is for a blood glucose level of 4–7 mmol/L before and during pregnancy.

Prescribe 5 mg/day folic acid prepregnancy and continue until 12 weeks' gestation. Check her rubella immunity status.

Offer her dietary advice. Encourage her to eat a diet with high levels of complex carbohydrates, soluble fibre and vitamins and reduced levels of saturated fats. Advise her on how to lose weight if her BMI is >27 kg/m² and also give general advice such as smoking cessation and reducing alcohol intake.

Carry out a retinal and renal assessment by way of fundoscopy, urine microalbuminuria and renal function tests. The risk of pre-eclampsia is increased with the presence of microalbuminuria or proteinuria.

Obstetrics and Gynaecology: Clinical Cases Uncovered.
By M. Cruickshank and A. Shetty. Published 2009 by Blackwell Publishing. ISBN 978-1-4051-8671-1.

Reinforce the idea that she will require additional time and effort to manage her diabetes in pregnancy and encourage frequent contact with health care professionals. The risk of diabetes in her child would be around 2–3%.

Ms Kumar's HbA1c is 13% with high fasting and postprandial sugars. She has no ketones or protein in her urine. She is immune to rubella and the renal function tests are normal. There is no evidence of retinopathy. She is on enalapril for hypertension, which is changed to methyldopa. She is advised to continue the progesterone-only pill until the blood sugar levels are optimized and HbA1c <6.1%. Lifestyle advice is also given. A follow-up visit in 3 months' time shows good glycaemic control with normalization of HbA1c. She stops the contraceptive pill and hopes to conceive soon. She is taking 5 mg folic acid.

Angiotensin converting enzyme (ACE) inhibitors should be stopped before or soon after confirming pregnancy as they may cause oligohydramniosis, renal failure and hypotension in the fetus. Retinopathy should be treated prior to pregnancy.

Women with glomerular filtration rates <45 mL/min and/or proteinuria >5 g/day during pregnancy should be offered consultation with a nephrologist. Pregnancy in women with severe nephropathy should be discouraged because of the poor outcome associated with it both to the women and the fetus.

Ms Kumar asks about the effects of diabetes on pregnancy and the fetus and also the effects of pregnancy on diabetes.

How would you counsel her in this regard?
Effects of pregnancy on diabetes

Increasing doses of insulin would be required as pregnancy progresses because of physiological insulin resistance and decreased glucose tolerance as a result of anti-insulin hormones secreted by the placenta.

During pregnancy, hypoglycaemic unawareness and severe hypoglycaemia are common and diabetic ketoacidosis can develop more rapidly. Diabetic retinal and renal disease can deteriorate during pregnancy.

The incidence of worsening chronic hypertension or pregnancy-induced hypertension and/or pre-eclampsia is high (varying from 40% to 73% across series) in women with both incipient and overt nephropathy.

Effects of diabetes on pregnancy

There is an increased likelihood of:
- Pre-eclampsia
- Macrosomia, polyhydramnios and shoulder dystocia
- Caesarean section, operative vaginal delivery
- Worsening nephropathy and superimposed pre-eclampsia resulting in an increase in iatrogenic preterm delivery
- Infections

Box 21.1 Classification of diabetes complicating pregnancy

- Pregestational
- Type 1 (insulin-dependent)
- Type 2 (non-insulin-dependent)
- Gestational diabetes

Box 21.2 White's classification of type 1 diabetes

Class	Age of onset (years)	Duration (years)	Vascular disease	Therapy
A	Any	Any	None	A1-diet only
B	Over 20	<10	None	Insulin
C	10–19	10–19	None	Insulin
D	Before 10	>20	Benign retinopathy	Insulin
F	Any	Any	Nephropathy	Insulin
R	Any	Any	Proliferative retinopathy	Insulin
H	Any	Any	Heart disease	Insulin

Box 21.3 Gestational diabetes mellitus

Definition

Carbohydrate intolerance of variable severity with onset or first recognized during the present pregnancy. This definition will include women with abnormal glucose tolerance that reverts to normal after delivery, and a small number of women with undiagnosed type 1 or type 2 diabetes

Screening for gestational diabetes in women with risk factors is recommended if

- BMI >30 kg/m^2
- Previous macrosomic baby >4.5 kg
- Previous gestational diabetes
- Family history of diabetes (first degree relative with type 1 or type 2 diabetes)

- Women from high risk ethnic group – South Asian, Afro-Caribbean, Chinese

Diagnosis of gestational diabetes

In women with risk factors, a 2-hour 75 g oral glucose tolerance test at around 24–28 weeks should be used to diagnose GDM. If there has been a previous history of GDM, an OGTT at 16–18 weeks, and if normal, repeated again at 28 weeks is recommended. The criteria recommended for diagnosis of GDM are fasting venous plasma glucose >5.5 mmol/L or >9 mmol/L 2 hours after OGTT

A diagnosis of GDM identifies women at increased risk of developing type 2 diabetes in future

Effects of diabetes on the fetus and neonate

There is an increased likelihood of:

• Congenital malformation – the risk is related to the glycaemic control around the time of conception and directly related to the level of HbA1c. Sacral agenesis is a specific congenital abnormality associated with diabetes. Congenital heart defect, skeletal abnormalities and neural tube defects are also more common.

• Spontaneous miscarriage.

• Unexplained fetal death *in utero*, highest after 36 weeks resulting from hypoxia in the presence of hyperglycaemia and lactic acidosis.

• Perinatal and neonatal mortality (increased by 5- to 10-fold).

• Macrosomia, defined as birth weight >4.5 kg or >90th centile for gestational age (seen especially with poor diabetic control).

In the neonate:

• Respiratory distress syndrome

• Hypoglycaemia

• Polycythaemia and jaundice

• Hypocalcaemia and hypomagnesaemia

• Hypertrophic cardiomyopathy

KEY POINT

Gestational diabetes mellitus (GDM) is associated with increased perinatal mortality and morbidity, but to a lesser degree than pre-existing diabetes.

There is no increased risk of congenital abnormality rate except in those with hyperglycaemia in first trimester or unrecognized diabetes predating pregnancy.

GDM is associated with an increased risk of macrosomia and pre-eclampsia.

Ms Kumar also wishes to know the target blood glucose ranges for pregnancy.

The target range to aim for during pregnancy is a fasting blood glucose between 3.5 and 5.9 mmol/L and 1-hour postprandial blood glucose <7.8 mmol/L during pregnancy.

She should be advised of the risks of hypoglycaemia and the difficulties in always being aware of this in pregnancy, particularly in the first trimester. She should be provided with glucagon injections and herself and her partner and family should be instructed in its use. Ketone

---

Box 21.4 Medical management of gestational diabetes

• Management with diet initially with reduced fat, increased fibre and regulation of carbohydrate intake

• If, after nutritional advice, pre- and postprandial glucose levels are normal and there is no evidence of excessive fetal growth, manage as a normal pregnancy

• Intensive management with diet and/or insulin if macrosomia is suspected or if blood glucose levels are in the range for established diabetes

• Newer sulphonylureas and metformin may be used as alternatives to insulin in GDM

---

testing strips and advice regarding testing for ketonuria or ketonaemia if hyperglycaemic or unwell should be offered.

Twice-daily mixed short-acting and intermediate-acting insulin should be changed to a four times daily basal bolus regimen (three premeal injections of fast acting insulin and nocturnal intermediate acting insulin) as it allows maximum flexibility in altering insulin dosage to compensate for the increased requirements of pregnancy and is also associated with fewer instances of neonatal and maternal hypoglycaemia.

Those with Type 2 diabetes require treatment with insulin even if well-controlled with oral hypoglycaemics. Conversion to insulin could be carried out either before or in early pregnancy. Oral hypoglycaemics (both sulphonylureas and biguanides) are traditionally avoided in pregnancy because they cross the placenta and there is a theoretical risk of fetal hypoglycaemia. However, there is some evidence that continuing metformin in pregnancy may be beneficial.

Women with diabetes who are pregnant should be offered early referral to a joint diabetes and antenatal clinic (Box 21.4).

Ms Kumar sees her GP with 9 weeks' amenorrhoea and is delighted to have a positive pregnancy test. The GP refers her to the combined obstetric and diabetic clinic for a booking visit.

How would you manage her at the booking visit?

• Confirm viability of pregnancy and gestational age by ultrasound

• Offer information, advice and support for optimizing glycaemic control

• Take a clinical history to establish the extent of diabetes-related complications
• Review medications for diabetes and its complications
• Offer retinal and renal assessment if these have not been undertaken in the previous 12 months
• Discuss antenatal screening tests

Ms Kumar has a normal booking scan which shows a single intrauterine live pregnancy of 10 weeks' gestation. She wishes to undergo mid-trimester serum screening for Down's syndrome. Her glycaemic control is optimal with normal HbA1c levels. Both retinal assessment and renal function tests are normal. Her blood pressure is 130/80 mmHg on 250 mg methyldopa twice daily. There is no proteinuria or ketonuria.

Regular growth scans every 4 weeks from 28 weeks onwards, to detect macrosomia and polyhydramnios is advised. Detailed retinal examination in early pregnancy and at least once in each trimester thereafter according to the severity of any retinopathy detected is also advised.

Women with nephropathy require regular monitoring of renal function (serum urea creatinine) and quantification of proteinuria (24-hour protein excretion, protein:creatinine ratio).

Her serum screening for Down's syndrome is low risk. The anomaly and the fetal cardiac scan are normal. Glycaemic control remains optimal. She presents at 29 weeks with painful contractions every 3–4 minutes. Abdominal examination confirms the fetus to be cephalic, the uterus to be non-tender and the uterine contractions strong every 1–3 minutes. The cardiotocogram (CTG) is normal. Vaginal examination shows the cervix to be 1 cm long, 1 cm dilated and soft. There are no symptoms of urinary tract infection and the urine dipstick test is normal.

What is your diagnosis and how would you manage her?

The diagnosis is preterm labour. She would need a midstream specimen of urine (MSSU) for culture and sensitivity, high vaginal swab (HVS), full blood count (FBC), C-reactive protein (CRP) and urea and electrolytes (U&E).

Steroids (12 mg betamethasone, 24 hours apart) for fetal lung maturation would be indicated, and tocolysis with atosiban (see Case 19) should be considered to allow for completion of the course of steroids. Additional

insulin cover either by way of a sliding scale or subcutaneous insulin, according to an agreed protocol, is indicated as both steroids and atosiban can worsen glycaemic control.

She receives both the doses of betamethasone IM. All investigations are normal. The contractions settle and she is discharged home after 3 days in hospital. For the rest of the pregnancy her glycaemic control remains good and BP well controlled with methyldopa. Induction of labour is planned for 38 weeks + 5 days' gestation.

KEY POINT

Plan delivery by way of induction or caesarean section between 38 and 39 weeks, although in well-controlled diabetes, in the absence of macrosomia or hypertension, the pregnancy may be allowed to progress to 40 weeks. Pregnancy should not be allowed to continue beyond 40 weeks in women with pre-existing diabetes.

If GDM is well controlled with normal fetal growth, await spontaneous labour.

Ms Kumar is induced with vaginal prostaglandin E$_2$. She then has an artificial rupture of membranes followed by Syntocinon augmentation. The fetus is monitored with continuous CTG.

How would you manage her in labour?

Commence an insulin sliding scale from the onset of established labour. Monitor capillary blood glucose on an hourly basis and aim to maintain this between 4 and 7 mmol/L.

KEY POINT

An insulin sliding scale should be started at the onset of spontaneous labour, prior to caesarean section or when glycaemic control is difficult to maintain (e.g. while receiving steroids or atosiban).

An infusion of 500 mL 10% glucose with 10 mmol KCL, is commenced at 100 mL/hour via a controlled infusion pump. An intravenous insulin infusion, 50 units Humulin soluble insulin made up to 50 mL with normal saline, is started at an initial rate of 2 units/hour (2 mL/hour) by syringe pump.

Blood glucose is measured regularly using blood glucose measuring strips with the aim of maintaining it at 4–7 mmol/L by varying the insulin infusion rate.

Ms Kumar has an emergency lower segment caesarean section for failure to progress at 7cm. The baby weighs 4.2kg with a good Apgar score. The procedure is uncomplicated, with a blood loss of 470mL.

What would be the postpartum management?

The rate of insulin infusion should be halved following delivery of the placenta, as her requirements for insulin reduce postpartum. Once she is eating normally, subcutaneous insulin should be recommenced at the prepregnancy dosage.

The baby should be fed as soon as possible after birth (within 30 minutes) and then at frequent intervals (2–3 hours) until feeding maintains blood glucose levels >2.0mmol/L. The baby should have blood glucose testing after feeding to rule out neonatal hypoglycaemia.

KEY POINT

In women with GDM on insulin, following delivery of placenta, the insulin should be stopped. Women with GDM should undergo formal 75g oral glucose tolerance test (OGTT) 6 weeks following delivery to exclude diabetes present outside of pregnancy. They should be counselled regarding the risks of future diabetes and receive lifestyle advice concerning exercise, diet and reduced fat intake.

Ms Kumar makes a good postnatal recovery. She is commenced on her prepregnancy dosage of insulin with which her sugars are well controlled. Both mother and baby are discharged on day 5 postoperatively and a follow-up appointment arranged for the diabetic clinic. She has a Depo-Provera injection for contraception before discharge.

CASE REVIEW

Ms Kumar, who had IDDM, presented appropriately to the prepregnancy clinic for advice which gave an opportunity to optimize her glycaemic control, stress the importance of optimizing glucose control and its effects on the fetus and pregnancy. The antihypertensive enalapril was stopped and was replaced with methyldopa. Folic acid 5mg was also started. Prepregnancy renal function and retinal examination were also performed. She came off contraception and conceived once the HbA1c was normalized.

Antenatal care was in the combined clinic where she was seen by a team comprising a diabetologist, obstetrician, dietitian, diabetic nurse and midwife. Antenatally, she required increasing doses of insulin with very good glycaemic control. She had regular growth scans which showed fetal growth to be on the 95th centile with polyhydramnios.

Labour was induced at 38+ weeks. She was commenced on insulin sliding scale in established labour to maintain her blood sugars. As a result of failure to progress in labour, an emergency lower segment caesarean section was performed. The sliding scale continued until she could eat following the caesarean section, when she went back on to her prepregnancy regimen of insulin.

KEY POINTS

- An experienced multidisciplinary team led by a named obstetrician and physician should provide comprehensive maternity care
- Pregnancy should be planned and good contraceptive advice and prepregnancy counselling are essential
- Dietary advice should be made available, and should encourage diets with high levels of complex carbohydrates, soluble fibre and vitamins, and reduced levels of saturated fats
- All women with diabetes should be prescribed prepregnancy folate supplementation (5 mg), continuing up to 12 weeks' gestation. Before and during pregnancy, women with diabetes should aim to have blood glucose levels between 4 and 7 mmol/L
- Fundal examination prior to conception and during each trimester is advised. More frequent assessment may be required in those with poor glycaemic control or hypertension
- ACE inhibitors should be avoided as they may adversely affect the fetus. Appropriate antihypertensive agents that may be used during pregnancy include methyldopa, labetalol and nifedipine
- Women with insulin-requiring diabetes in pregnancies that are otherwise progressing normally should be assessed at 38 weeks' gestation to ensure delivery by 40 weeks
- Women with diabetes should be delivered in consultant-led maternity units with access to a senior physican, obstetrician and neonatologist
- The progress of labour should be monitored as for other high risk women, including continuous electronic fetal monitoring
- Intravenous insulin and dextrose should be administered as necessary to maintain blood glucose levels between 4 and 7 mmol/L
- Early feeding is advised to avoid neonatal hypoglycaemia and to stimulate lactation

Further reading

NICE Clinical Guideline CG63. *Diabetes in pregnancy: management of diabetes and its complications from pre-conception to the postnatal period.* March 2008.

A 32-year-old woman with a fetus in the breech position at 37 weeks' gestation

Mrs Alvares is 37 weeks' pregnant, this is her first pregnancy. She comes to the antenatal clinic as she saw her community midwife last week and although all was well her midwife thought her baby may be breech. Her routine antenatal check is reassuring but the baby does seem to be in a breech presentation.

What will you tell Mrs Alvares?

Instead of the normal head down position her baby seems to be presenting 'bottom first'. This is not uncommon, about 20% of babies are breech at 28 weeks but they usually turn on their own so only about 3–4% are breech at term.

The baby may still turn on its own but if it does not the options include turning the baby to face head down (external cephalic version [ECV]), elective caesarean section or vaginal breech delivery.

What investigations are required?

An ultrasound scan should be performed to confirm the presentation. In some cases a baby will adopt a breech position because of a fetal or uterine abnormality, reduced liquor volume or placenta praevia and these conditions need to be excluded.

Mrs Alvares has a scan which confirms that her baby is breech with flexed legs. The baby is normally grown and has a normal liquor volume. The placenta is normally located and there is no obvious uterine or fetal abnormality to account for the breech presentation (Fig. 22.1; Box 22.1).

What information should you give Mrs Alvares about delivery?

She should be informed that planned caesarean section

carries a reduced perinatal mortality and early neonatal morbidity for babies with a breech presentation at term compared with a planned vaginal birth. There is no evidence that the long-term health of babies with a breech presentation delivered at term is influenced by how the baby is born.

She should be advised that planned caesarean section for breech presentation carries a small increase in serious immediate complications for her compared with planned vaginal birth. It does not carry any additional risk to her long-term health outside pregnancy. The long-term effect of planned caesarean section on future pregnancy outcomes is uncertain.

Mrs Alvares would prefer not to have a cesarean section but is worried about the risk to the baby of a vaginal breech delivery. She remembers that you mentioned that it might be possible to turn the baby to face head down and would like some further information about this.

What will you tell her?

The procedure called external cephalic version (ECV) involves external manipulation of the baby through the maternal abdomen to turn the baby to a cephalic presentation. It should be performed after 36 weeks with a first baby and after 37 weeks in parous women. The success rate is aproximately 40% with a first baby and approximately 60% in parous women. If it is successful, less than 5% of babies will turn back to breech.

The risks to the baby include acute fetal distress, spontaneous rupture of the fetal membranes and placental abruption which may require emergency cesarean section but these occur very uncommonly. It can cause a significant amount of maternal discomfort.

She thinks she would like to have an ECV performed. An appointment is made for the following day and she returns to labour ward. She wants to know exactly what will happen.

Obstetrics and Gynaecology: Clinical Cases Uncovered.
By M. Cruickshank and A. Shetty. Published 2009 by Blackwell Publishing. ISBN 978-1-4051-8671-1.

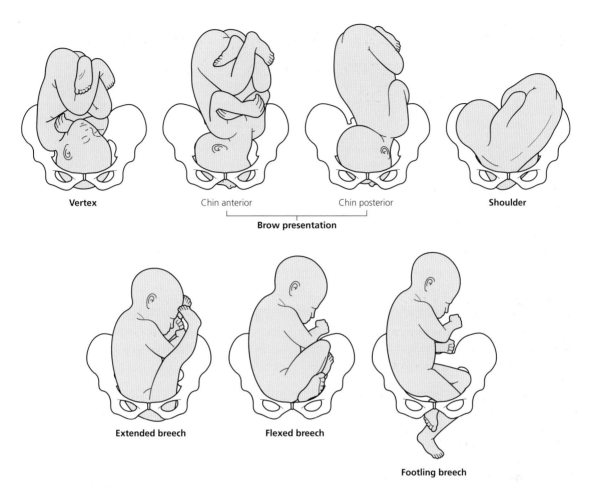

Vertex   Chin anterior   Chin posterior   Shoulder

Brow presentation

Extended breech   Flexed breech

Footling breech

Figure 22.1 Fetal malpresentation.

Box 22.1 Fetal malpresentation

By 37 weeks >95% of babies will be in a longitudinal lie and vertex presentation. The remainder will be breech, face or brow presentations (also longitudinal lie) and oblique, transverse or unstable (variable) lies. Of these the breech and face presentations are, at least in theory, able to be delivered vaginally.

The risks of malpresentation are related to obstructed labour and the risk of uterine rupture secondary to prolonged contractions without any prospect of delivery. The other major risk with a non-longitudinal lie is of umbilical cord or a limb prolapsing through the cervix when the fetal membranes rupture. In view of this, women with non-longitudinal or unstable lies will normally be managed as inpatients from about 36 weeks until delivery or until the fetal lie stabilizes.

Maternal causes of malpresentation include uterine abnormality (e.g. fibroids or a placenta praevia) and high parity also increases the risk. Fetal causes include multiple pregnancy, reduced liquor volume or fetal abnormality preventing a cephalic presentation.

What would you discuss with her?

She will be monitored by cardiotocogram (CTG) to check the baby's heart rate before the procedure is commenced. An ultrasound scan will be performed to check baby is still breech and to identify where the fetal back is posi-tioned. Tocolysis (uterine relaxation) will be offered as it has been proven to improve success rates (usually by IV or subcutaneous beta-sympathomimetics).

She will be positioned in a slightly head down position (to try to elevate the breech out of the pelvis) with a

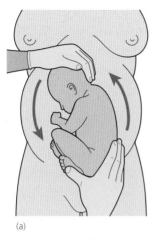
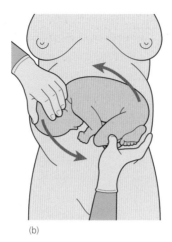
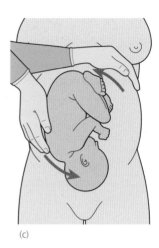

(a)   (b)   (c)

Figure 22.2 External cephalic version.

wedge under her right hip (to prevent aorto-caval compression from the pregnant uterus when lying flat). Pressure will be used on the maternal abdomen to try to elevate the breech out of the pelvis and turn the baby through a forward or backward roll to a cephalic presentation. Ultrasound can be used to guide the procedure.

Following the procedure, whether successful or not, she will be put back on the CTG to make sure the baby is healthy.

RCOG guidelines recommend that women undergoing ECV do not need to be prepared for caesarean section as the chance of this being required as an emergency is very small (Fig. 22.2).

There are three attempts at ECV with tocolysis but unfortunately the baby remains breech. The post-ECV CTG is reassuring. Mrs Alvares is sure she does not want a vaginal breech delivery and would like some further information about caesarean section.

What will you tell her?

To reduce the risks of breathing problems in the baby, elective caesarean sections are usually carried out after 39 weeks. She would normally be admitted on the morning of her section. She would be asked to fast from midnight the night before and take some antacid tablets (to reduce the risks of aspiration if general anaesthetic became necessary).

Prior to the caesarean section, the lie of the baby would be checked on ultrasound to confirm it was still in the breech position. If it was found to be head down she would be advised to go home to await normal labour. She would normally receive a spinal anaesthetic for her section as this is associated with reduced risks to mother and baby, and would allow her to be awake to see her baby at birth.

Once her anaesthetic is working a catheter will be placed in her bladder and her section will be carried out through a 'bikini-line' incision. The baby and placenta are delivered through the incision and then the uterus and layers of the abdominal wall are repaired, the procedure usually takes 45–60 minutes. Afterwards she will be given painkillers as necessary and will usually be fit to go home after 3–5 days.

Having a baby, either vaginally or by caesarean section, carries a risk of excess bleeding sometimes requiring blood transfusion and a risk of infection. Caesarean section carries an increased risk of thrombosis (DVT) and damage to bladder and ureters compared with vaginal delivery. In order to minimize these risks antibiotic prophylaxis is given during the procedure and thromboprophylaxis is given postnatally.

The positive and negative effects of caesarean section have been extensively investigated. The NICE guideline on caesarean section summarizes these in one of its appendices.

Mrs Alvares is happy with the explanation and is booked for an elective section at 39 weeks. She is admitted as planned and, as the baby remains in a breech presentation, has an uncomplicated elective section. She has a female baby in good condition weighing 3.24 kg and is fit for discharge after 3 days.

CASE REVIEW

Mrs Alvares has a breech presentation of the fetus diagnosed at 37 weeks' gestation. A placenta praevia, abnomalities of liquor volume and uterine abnormality are ruled out by an ultrasound examination and she is counselled about an external cephalic version to manually turn the baby to a cephalic position so that she could attempt a vaginal delivery. Following consent for the procedure, she is given tocolysis to increase the likelihood of it being successful; however, ECV fails and the fetus remains in a breech position.

She then opts for an elective caesarean section as mode of delivery after being counselled that a planned caesarean section carries a small reduced perinatal mortality and early neonatal morbidity. Her caesarean section proceeds without event and she makes a good postoperative recovery. In a subsequent pregnancy, provided there are no other concerns and the baby is in a cephalic position, she could opt for a trial of vaginal delivery.

Malpresentation at term is associated with increased perinatal morbidity and mortality. When faced with this problem the options include vaginal delivery of a non-vertex presentation, attempting to convert the fetal lie to a vertex presentation or delivery of the baby by caesarean section depending on the malpresentation involved. Decisions regarding the most appropriate course of action should be made in conjunction with the parents ensuring that they are fully informed of all the available evidence regarding risks, benefits and potential outcomes of the various options.

KEY POINTS

- While malpresentations are seen more often at earlier gestations, this reduces to <5% at term (>37 weeks)
- A low lying placenta, fibroids in the lower segment of the uterus, polyhydramnios are some of the predisposing factors for fetal malposition
- The risks with an oblique or a transverse or an unstable fetal lie (where there is no fetal part fixed in the pelvis) include one of cord prolapse in case of rupture of membranes. In view of this risk (which would necessitate an emergency delivery), these women should ideally be managed as inpatients after 36–37 weeks (until delivery) as long as the malposition remains
- An ECV should be offered to women with a malposition at >36 weeks' gestation, once other risk factors such as a low lying placenta have been ruled out
- Tocolysis improves the success rate of an ECV, as does being multiparous

Further reading

RCOG Green Top Clinical Guideline (no 20a). *External cephalic version and reducing the incidence of breech presentation.* December 2006.

Case 23   A 26-year-old woman with a history of one previous caesarean section booking at the antenatal clinic

Mrs Mclean is a 26-year-old woman, booking at the antenatal clinic in her second pregnancy at 13 weeks' gestation. Her booking scan is normal. Her first pregnancy culminated in an emergency caesarean section 2 years ago.

What other information would you need?

The details of her previous labour and operation.

Indication for the previous caesarean section

Was it for a recurrent or non-recurrent indication? There are very few recurrent indications (e.g. severely contracted pelvis). Most caesarean sections are for non-recurrent indications which include breech presentation, fetal distress and non-progress of labour.

Type of caesarean section (lower or upper uterine segment caesarean section)

Most caesarean sections are performed through the lower segment of the uterus (Fig. 23.1). The few indications for an upper segment (classic) caesarean section include one that may need to be performed at a very preterm gestation where the lower segment is not well formed, for a transverse lie with rupture of membranes and no liquor to manipulate the fetus or for a major placenta praevia.

Intraoperative or postoperative complications

Intraoperative complications include extension of the lower uterine segment incision or injury to the bladder, bowel or increased bleeding or uterine atony at caesarean section. Postoperative complications include infections (endometritis, pelvic infection, superficial wound infection or of other systems including chest infections) or thrombosis.

Mrs Mclean has had an uncomplicated lower segment caesarean at 7 cm cervical dilatation for fetal distress. The postoperative period was uneventful. The birth weight of her son was 3.7 kg.

How would you counsel her?

She should be given the choice of trial of labour (vaginal birth after caesarean section [VBAC]) or elective repeat caesarean section (ERCS) as she has had a lower segment caesarean section for a non-recurrent indication. Maternal and perinatal benefits and risks of VBAC and ERCS should be discussed.

Successful VBAC occurs in 72–76% of women attempting it, with a 24–28% chance of requiring an emergency caesarean section. Successful VBAC has the advantage of shorter hospital stay, quick recovery and good chance of vaginal delivery in subsequent pregnancies. Also, the risk of the baby having respiratory problems after birth is reduced with VBAC.

VBAC carries a risk of uterine rupture of 22–74/10,000 with one previous caesarean section (Box 23.1). There is no risk of uterine rupture in women undergoing ERCS. The risks of scar rupture with two previous caesarean sections is not clearly known (approximately 92/10,000). There is also an additional 1% risk of blood transfusion, endometritis and 2–3/10,000 additional risk of birth-related perinatal death with VBAC when compared with ERCS. ERCS carries the risk of bleeding, infection, thromboembolism, operative injury and may increase the risk of serious complications in future pregnancies.

> **KEY POINT**
>
> *Timing of elective caesarean section.* Caesarean section should be carried out after 39 weeks to decrease the risk of neonatal respiratory distress syndrome.

Obstetrics and Gynaecology: Clinical Cases Uncovered.
By M. Cruickshank and A. Shetty. Published 2009 by Blackwell Publishing. ISBN 978-1-4051-8671-1.

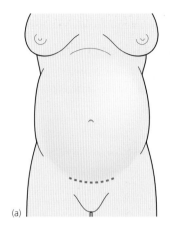

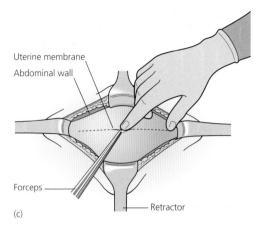

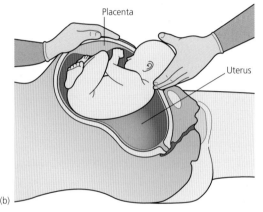

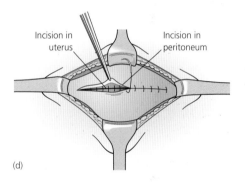

Figure 23.1 Lower segment caesarean section.

Box 23.1 Contraindications to VBAC

- Previous one classic (upper segment) caesarean section
- Three or more previous caesarean sections
- Previous uterine rupture or scar dehiscence

Mrs Mclean fully understands the advantages and disadvantages of VBAC and ERCS. She is very keen for a vaginal delivery at home.

What would you advise her?

She should be advised to deliver in the hospital as VBAC should be conducted in a suitably staffed and equipped delivery suit, with continuous intrapartum and electronic fetal monitoring with immediate access to caesarean section, neonatal resuscitation and on-site blood transfusion.

Mrs Mclean does not want any risk to herself or the baby and now wishes a VBAC in the hospital. She wants to know the options for pain relief in labour.

What pain relief options are available to her in labour?

She has the option of using Entonox, morphine, transcutaneous electrical nerve stimulation (TENS) or epidural. Epidural analgesia is not contraindicated with VBAC.

Further antenatal appointments are with the community midwife. She has the serum screening for Down's syndrome at 16 weeks which puts her in the low risk category and her 20-week detailed anomaly scan is normal.

When would you wish to see her in the antenatal clinic and what investigation would you arrange before the review?

An antenatal review around 36 weeks gestation to discuss her decision about mode of delivery and evaluate any risk factors that would exclude a VBAC would be indicated. If at her 20-week scan the placenta has been documented to be implanted anteriorly on the uterus, she would need an ultrasound to rule out a low lying placenta (see Case 17; previous caesarean section is a risk factor for a low lying placenta which may also be adherent if implanted over the old scar).

Mrs Mclean is seen by the community midwife at 24, 28 and 32 weeks. The ultrasound at 36 weeks confirms the placenta to be fundal and anterior with normal growth and liquor. Her final decision about the mode of delivery is to have a vaginal delivery. Rest of her antenatal care is with the community midwife who refers her to the antenatal clinic at 41 weeks (postdates) to discuss induction of labour.

What options does she have?
She has the option of ERCS or induction of labour (artificial rupture of membranes with oxytocin augmentation or prostaglandin cervical ripening, depending on cervical Bishop's score) at 41–42 weeks.

What advice would you give her about induction of labour?
There is two- to threefold increased risk of uterine rupture and 1.5-fold increased risk of caesarean section in induced or augmented labours compared to spontaneous labour. There is higher risk of uterine rupture with induction of labour with prostaglandins than with non-prostaglandins (2.4% vs 0.8%.).

KEY POINT

The decision to induce and the method chosen should be consultant led.

On discussing the options Mrs Mclean opts for induction of labour. Vaginal examination shows the cervix to be 2 cm dilated, 1 cm long (50–60% effaced), soft, mid-position and the station of the presenting part at 2 cm above the ischial spine (Bishop's cervical score of 7 'favorable cervix'; see Case 14).

A membrane sweep is performed and she is booked for artificial rupture of membranes and oxytocin augmentation at 10 days past the expected date of delivery. She presents to labour ward the next day with spontaneous rupture of membranes and contractions.

How would you manage her initially?
• Intravenous access, full blood count (FBC) and group and save
• Abdominal examination and cardiotocograph (CTG) monitoring
• Sterile speculum examination to confirm rupture of membranes
• Cervical assessment to determine the stage of labour

Two to three mild to moderate uterine contractions are felt every 10 minutes. The CTG is reassuring. Vaginal examination shows the cervix to be 4 cm dilated, fully effaced with the presenting part 2 cm above the spines. Clear liquor is seen draining and the membranes are confirmed to be ruptured.

What should be the subsequent management?
• Continuous CTG monitoring
• Regular assessment of uterine contractions
• Careful serial cervical assessment, preferably by the same person, to ensure there is adequate progress in cervical dilatation and descent of the fetal head in the maternal pelvis
• Monitor for signs of uterine rupture (Box 23.2)

Subsequent vaginal examination, 6 hours from the initial examination, shows the cervix dilatation still at 4 cm, with the presenting part at –2 station in an occipito-transverse position. Two mild contractions are felt every 2 minutes. There are no signs of scar rupture. After appropriate counselling (to reinforce the risks of scar rupture with augmentation of labour with oxytocin), in view of the

---

Box 23.2 Concerning clinical features of utering rupture

• Abnormal CTG
• Severe abdominal pain, especially if persisting between contractions
• Chest pain or shoulder tip pain, sudden onset of shortness of breath
• Acute onset of scar tenderness
• Abnormal vaginal bleeding or haematuria
• Cessation of previously effective uterine contractions
• Maternal tachycardia, hypotension or shock
• Loss of the station of the presenting part in the maternal pelvis

> **Box 23.3 Classification of urgency of caesarean section**
>
> **Emergency caesarean section**
> Immediate threat to the life of the mother or the fetus (delivery should be accomplished within 30 minutes), e.g. placenta abruption, cord prolapse, profound or prolonged fetal bradycardia
>
> **Urgent caesarean section**
> Maternal or fetal compromise that is not immediately life-threatening, e.g. none or slow progress of labour where the mother and fetus are in good condition
>
> **Scheduled caesarean section**
> No maternal or fetal compromise, but needs early delivery, e.g. breech presentation at term with ruptured membranes, but not in labour
>
> **Elective caesarean section**
> Delivery timed to suit woman or staff, e.g. planned caesarean section for breech presentation at term or for previous two caesarean sections

non-progress of labour, oxytocin intravenous infusion is commenced for augmentation of labour at Mrs Mclean's request. Repeat vaginal examination 4 hours after regular contractions shows no change in the cervix or in the position or station of the head despite strong and regular contractions. The CTG is reassuring.

What would you advise her now?

In view of failure to progress despite strong and regular contractions, she should be advised an urgent caesarean section (Box 23.3).

Mrs Mclean consents to go ahead with a caesarean section. She also makes a request for sterilization at the time of caesarean section.

What would you advise her about sterilization and what preoperative assessment should be performed?

She should be advised that for sterilization to be performed at the time of caesarean section, counselling and agreement should have been given at least 1 week prior to the procedure, and should not be not be considered for the first time in an emergency situation. She should have had time to consider the permanence of the procedure, the failure rate of about 1 in 300, the small risk of future ectopic pregnancies and menstrual irregularities, and the alternative methods of reversible contraception.

Preoperative assessment involves:
- Checking haemoglobin level on FBC
- Prescribing of prophylactic antibiotic (one intraoperative dose of cephalosporin or augmentin)
- Assessing thromboembolic risk
- Siting an indwelling catheter
- Offer antiemetic, antacid and H_2 receptor analogues
- Anaesthetic review – offer regional anaesthesia and discuss postoperative pain relief

Mrs Mclean has an uncomplicated urgent lower segment caesarean section under spinal anaesthesia. A male baby weighing 3.8 kg with good Apgar scores of 9/10 and 9/10 at 1 and 5 minutes is delivered. She receives intraoperative prophylactic antibiotics. The total blood loss is 780 mL. She is prescribed a prophylactic dose of dalteparin postoperatively.

What postoperative care should she receive?

- Offer patient-controlled opioid analgesia (PCA) or oral opioids for pain
- Offer a non-steroidal anti-inflammatory drug (NSAID) to reduce the need for opioids
- Additional support to start breastfeeding as soon as possible
- Urinary catheter could be removed 12 hours after spinal or last top-up of epidural analgesia
- She should eat and drink when hungry or thirsty
- If she recovers well and remains apyrexial she could be discharged home on the second or third postoperative day with follow-up by the community midwife
- Discuss the reasons for caesarean section and implications before discharge
- Discuss contraception

Mrs Mclean makes a good recovery postnatally and is discharged home on the third postoperative day. Her haemoglobin at discharge is 98 g/L and she is commenced on oral ferrous sulphate tablets. On discussing the contraceptive options, she opts for an Implanon implant which could be inserted by the GP or in the family planning clinic. In any subsequent pregnancy, because of her history of two previous caesarean sections, an elective caesarean section is an option for her, although if she were very keen she might be able to opt for another VBAC (understanding the risks especially of scar rupture), especially if she labours spontaneously.

CASE REVIEW

Mrs Mclean, who has a history of one previous caesarean section, opts for a VBAC after adequate counselling. Following a membrane sweep at 40+ weeks she goes into labour spontaneously but her uterine contractions are not very effective and there is slow progress in labour. After counselling regarding the increased risks of scar rupture with oxytocin, she wishes augmentation of contractions with an oxytocin infusion. She is closely monitored for signs of scar rupture throughout her labour. Her labour remains dystocic in spite of oxytocin and she has an urgent caesarean section for this indication.

Increasing rates of primary caesarean section have led to an increased proportion of the obstetric population who have a history of prior caesarean delivery. The National Caesarean Section Rate (CSR) in England was 21.3% in 2001 and the group contributing most to the overall CSR is that composed of women at term with a singleton cephalic pregnancy and a previous caesarean section.

Pregnant women with a previous section may be offered either planned VBAC or ERCS. The proportion of women who decline VBAC is, in turn, a significant determinant of overall rates of caesarean birth. Hence, these women should be counselled adequately antenatally. This counselling should include the statistics for success rates with a VBAC, the risks of scar rupture, both with spontaneous labour and induction/augmentation agents (prostaglandins, oxytocin), the need for CTG monitoring during labour and assessments for clinical signs of scar rupture, at a site where facilities for immediate caesarean section are available. The operative risks and the impact on her future obstetric career with a repeat caesarean section should also be discussed, and an informed choice regarding mode of delivery should ideally be made around 36–37 weeks' gestation. With increasing numbers of caesarean sections there is an increased risk of bleeding, placenta praevia and accreta, injury to bladder and bowel, ileus, of hysterectomy and the need for blood transfusion.

KEY POINTS

- There are very few recurrent indications for a caesarean section and the majority of women with one previous caesarean section should be able to have the choice of a VBAC in their next pregnancy
- Overall, the chances of a successful vaginal delivery with a VBAC are 72–76%, with the risk of scar rupture approximately 22–74/1000.

- The risks of scar rupture are two- to threefold greater with induced or augmented VBAC labours than with spontaneous labour. The risks are greatest where prostaglandin cervical ripening is used
- Continuous intrapartum care and CTG monitoring is recommended with VBAC to enable prompt detection of scar rupture

Further reading

NICE Clinical Guideline (no 13). *Caesarean section*. April 2004.
RCOG Green Top Guidelines (no. 45). *Birth after previous caesarean birth*. RCOG Press, London, February 2007.

A 29-year-old woman with vomiting in early pregnancy

Mrs Begum, a 29-year-old para 1, is referred to the assessment unit at the maternity hospital by her GP on account of persistent vomiting. She is approximately 7 weeks pregnant by dates, has been unable to keep anything down because of ongoing vomiting. She feels exhausted and unable to cope.

What differential diagnosis comes to your mind?

- Hyperemesis gravidarum
- Gastritis/gastroenteritis
- Urinary tract infection
- Other rare causes of vomiting, e.g. thyrotoxicosis, pancreatitis, Addison's disease, cholecystitis, hepatitis

---

KEY POINT

Hyperemesis gravidarum (HG) is defined as persistent vomiting in pregnancy, which leads to weight loss (>5% body mass) and ketosis. Although over 50% of pregnant women experience nausea and vomiting, HG affects 1% of pregnancies.

What would you like to elicit from the history?
Presenting complaints

- Duration, frequency and amount of vomiting
- Any heartburn, abdominal pain or diarrhoea
- Any urinary symptoms
- Mood changes

Obstetrics and Gynaecology: Clinical Cases Uncovered.
By M. Cruickshank and A. Shetty. Published 2009 by Blackwell
Publishing. ISBN 978-1-4051-8671-1.

Obstetric history

Details of previous pregnancy including a history of hyperemesis.

Past medical history including allergies

Any medical problems, e.g. pancreatitis, Addison's disease, hyperthyroidism

Family history

- Anybody else in the family with similar symptoms
- Is there a history of twins in the family?

Mrs Begum states that her nausea and vomiting started a week ago and has been getting progressively worse .She now feels sick all the time, is unable to keep any food down. She vomits small amounts approximately 10–12 times a day. She also admits to having some heartburn but denies any abdominal pain, diarrhoea or urinary symptoms. She has been feeling low and is unable to cope any more.

She has had one pregnancy in the past and her daughter, Ayesha, is now 2 years old. She has a history of two admissions early in her first pregnancy with intractable vomiting requiring intravenous fluids and antiemetics.

She gives no history of medical problems or allergies. She has non-identical twin brothers and reports that no one else in the family has experienced similar symptoms

---

KEY POINT

Hyperemesis gravidarum: onset is always in first trimester, commonly around 6–8 weeks.

What key features would you look for during physical examination?
General examination

- Signs of dehydration, e.g. dry skin and mouth, decreased skin turgor

Table 24.1 Clinical signs of dehydration.

Dehydration	Mild	Moderate	Severe
Skin turgor	Normal	Dry	Clammy
Buccal mucosa/lips	Moist	Dry	Parched/cracked
Pulse	Regular	Slightly increased	Increased, low volume
Urine output	Normal	Decreased	Anuric

- Pulse, blood pressure and temperature recording: tachycardia and postural hypotension suggest dehydration
- Assess mood – e.g. unkempt appearance, tearfulness

Routine systemic examination
To assess general health and exclude medical problems.

Mrs Begum is very tearful during the consultation. She appears tired and run down but not in any pain. Her skin and lips appear dry and there is tenting of her skin. Her pulse is 98 beats/minute, of low volume and she appears to have postural hypotension as indicated by lying and standing blood pressures. These vital parameters indicate that she is moderately dehydrated (Table 24.1). Systemic examination is unremarkable.

What would be the next step?
Obtain a sample of urine for dipstick analysis and urine pregnancy test
- Confirm pregnancy
- Increased specific gravity (dehydration)
- Presence of ketones (dehydration)
- Presence of nitrites/leucocytes/blood (may suggest urinary infection)

What investigations would you like to carry out?
Blood tests
- *Full blood count (FBC):* an increased haematocrit suggests haemoconcentration
- *Urea and electrolytes (U&E):* to look for hyponatraemia, hypokalaemia, low serum urea, hypochloraemic alkalosis
- *Liver function test (LFT):* LFTs are abnormal in up to 50% of women with HG

Box 24.1 Gestational hyperthyroidism

- Biochemical hyperthyroidism found in approximately 60% women with HG
- Self-limiting
- Patient clinically euthyroid
- Findings: ↑ free thyroxine (T4), ↓ thyroid stimulating hormone (TSH), negative thyroid antibodies
- Mechanism:
- human chorionic gonadotrophin (HCG) shares α subunit with TSH
- increased secretion of HCG/HCG oversensitive thyrotrophin receptors/secretion of variant of HCG
- Thyroid function tests provide an index of severity of HG
- More common in Asian women
- Rarely, Graves disease may present in pregnancy. The absence of TSH receptor, antiperoxidase, and antithyroglobulin autoantibodies supports the diagnosis of HG

- *Thyroid function test (TFT):* there may be transient biochemical hyperthyroidism (Box 24.1). Resolves without treatment by 18 weeks

Mid-stream sample of urine (MSSU)
To exclude urinary tract infection.

Pelvic ultrasound
- Confirms viability of the pregnancy
- Diagnoses twin gestation
- Excludes molar pregnancy

Mrs Begum is not anaemic but has a raised haematocrit along with hyponatraemia and hypokalaemia. Her LFTs and TFTs are within the normal range. A urine dipstick shows the presence of +++ ketones but is negative for nitrites, leucocytes and blood. The clinical features along with ketonuria and high urine specific gravity confirm dehydration. A pelvic ultrasound scan shows a dichorionic twin pregnancy of 7 weeks' gestation.

KEY POINT

Hyperemesis gravidarum is a diagnosis of exclusion. There is no single confirmatory test.

Thus, by a focused history, thorough clinical examination and relevant investigations other causes of vomiting are excluded. We can conclude that the likely diagnosis in Mrs Begum's case is that of hyperemesis gravidarum (Box 24.2).

Box 24.2 Pathophysiology of hyperemesis gravidarum

- Poorly understood, multifactorial
- Temporal relationship exists between level of human chorionic gonadotrophin (HCG) and severity of symptoms
- HCG peaks between 6 and 12 weeks coinciding with peak symptomatology
- Correlation with high HCG levels explains the increased incidence of HG in women with multiple pregnancy and hydatiform mole, both conditions associated with very high HCG levels
- Mechanical factors, e.g. decreased peristalsis and delayed gastric emptying, exacerbate the symptoms, but are not thought to be causative
- Psychological and behavioural theories exist but are not proven
- *Risk factors:* multiparity, past history of HG and eating disorder, multiple gestation, hydatiform mole
- Cigarette smoking and maternal age >30 years appear to be protective
- Evidence suggests infection with *Helicobacter pylori* may have a role

Box 24.3 Wernicke's encephalopathy

- Syndrome characterized by diplopic abnormal ocular movements, ataxia and confusion
- Precipitated by administration of IV dextrose/glucose in thiamine deficiency
- Residual impairment is common despite replacement
- Koraskoff's psychosis is characterized by amnesia, impaired ability to learn and confabulation (invented memories which are then taken as true because of gaps in the memory)

    ○ vitamin B_{12} and pyridoxine (B_6) – anaemia and neuropathy
- Thrombosis: the combination of dehydration and bed rest increase the risk of thrombosis
- Psychological problems: these are often underestimated

Fetal complications of hyperemesis gravidarum
- Severe HG is associated with low birth weight babies
- HG leading to Wernicke's encephalopathy is associated with fetal death in 40% of cases

The diagnosis is explained to Mrs Begum, who is very anxious, as her symptoms are much worse in her present pregnancy. She wonders if it could lead to any harm to herself or to her babies.

What are the complications associated with hyperemesis gravidarum?

Maternal complications of hyperemesis gravidarum
- Can lead to serious morbidity
- Mallory–Weiss tears of oesophagus and haematemesis because of persistent vomiting and retching
- Malnutrition
- Weight loss (up to10–20% of body mass), muscle wasting, weakness
- Hyponatraemia (plasma sodium <120 mmol/L):
  - ○ can cause lethargy, seizures and respiratory arrest
  - ○ severe hyponatraemia and its rapid correction can precipitate central pontine myelinolysis
- Vitamin deficiency:
  - ○ thiamine (B_1) – acute deficiency causes Wernicke's encephalopathy (Box 24.3) Residual impairment leads to Koraskoff's psychosis

How will you manage this woman, who has been diagnosed with hyperemesis at 7 weeks' gestation?

!RED FLAG
Management should be *early* and *aggressive* in view of increased risk of complications for mother and her fetus in the absence of treatment.

If tolerating orally the management includes rest, small but frequent carbohydrate meals along with adequate fluids orally. However, if she is unable to maintain hydration she should be admitted to hospital.

KEY POINT
Hyperemesis is a leading cause of hospitalization in early pregnancy.

Rehydration
Appropriate and adequate parentral fluid along with electrolyte replacement forms the mainstay of treatment. Rehydration with normal saline (0.9% saline, 150 mmol/L sodium) or Hartman's solution (0.6% saline, 132 mmol/L

sodium) is recommended. Add potassium chloride to fluid bags as directed by electrolyte levels. Check U&E daily while on intravenous fluids.

The patient should be weighed twice weekly for objective assessment of dehydration. Continue treatment until the patient can tolerate oral fluids and until test results show little or no ketones in the urine.

!RED FLAG

An infusion of dextrose-containing fluid can precipitate Wernicke's encephalopathy and is not recommended. Double strength saline should be avoided as rapid correction of hyponatraemia can cause central pontine myelinolysis.

Antiemetics

Antiemetics are recommended if rehydration and electrolyte replacement fail to improve the symptoms. Antiemetics should be prescribed on regular basis rather than as required. The intravenous or rectal route can be used initially and changed to oral route when tolerating orally (Table 24.2).

KEY POINT

The commonly used antiemetics, e.g. antihistamines, phenothiazines and dopamine antagonists, are not known to be associated with teratogenesis.

Table 24.2 Antiemetic agents.

Antihistamines	Cyclizine	H1 receptor antagonist
	Promethazine	Commonly used
		Good safety profile
Phenothiazines	Cholpromazine	Side-effects: drowsiness, extrapyramidal effects, oculogyric crisis
	Prochlorperazine	
Dopamine antagonist	Metcloptramide	Promotility agents
	Domperidone	Oculogyric crisis and extrapyramidal effects
Selective serotonin (5-HT3) antagonist	Ondansetron	Used for refractory HG
		Limited safety data
		Routine use not recommended

Thiamine (vitamin B$_1$) supplementation

Thiamine deficiency leads to Wernicke's encephalopathy. Thiamine supplementation is recommended in HG. If the patient is unable to tolerate this orally thiamine is administered as an infusion once a week.

Thromboprophylaxis

!RED FLAG

Dehydration, bed rest and reduced mobility and pregnancy are risk factors for thrombosis.

Women requiring hospitalization with HG should receive thromboprophylaxis. Prophylactic doses of low molecular weight heparin along with thromboembolic deterrent stockings (TEDS) should be used.

Psychological support

Emotional support from the medical team and the family aid the medical treatment. Psychotherapy, hypnotherapy and behavioural therapy have been reported to be of benefit.

Alternative therapies

Pyridoxine (vitamin B$_6$) has been reported to reduce the severity of nausea. Ginger, available as capsules, is helpful with nausea and vomiting with no apparent side-effects. Acupuncture is thought to reduce the symptoms and encourages weight gain.

Mrs Begum is commenced on 0.9% saline IV along with prochlorperazine (Stemetil) IM on a regular basis. She is given thromboprophylaxis in the form of low molecular weight heparin and TEDS. Her fluid therapy is monitored with daily U&E and urinary ketones. Thiamine is prescribed as a weekly infusion.

After 72 hours of aggressive fluid and regular antiemetic therapy Mrs Begum's condition shows marked improvement. Her symptoms settle and her urine is negative for ketones. She is commenced on oral antiemetics along with small frequent meals, which she tolerates well. She is keen to go home, as she feels much better. She is therefore discharged home with dietary advice on antiemetic therapy.

However, over the course of next few weeks she has several admissions with similar symptoms, which appear not to respond to conventional therapy. The doctor tells her she has 'refractory hyperemesis'.

PART 2: CASES

What would be the next step?
Ondensetron
This strong antiemetic is mostly used to treat nausea and vomiting postoperatively and following chemotherapy. It is an option for managing refractory HG. There are limited data on its safety in pregnancy.

Corticosteroids
Steroid therapy reported to be of benefit with dramatic improvement of symptoms with a significant reduction in readmission rates. Hydrocortisone IV followed by oral prednisolone are the preferred preparations. Dosage is gradually reduced to a maintenance dose of 5–10 mg/day by 20 weeks. No adverse fetal effects have been reported.

Total parentral nutrition and enteral feeding
This is expensive but can be life-saving in severe cases. Total parenteral nutrition (TPN) requires monitoring and protocol as can lead to infectious and metabolic complications.

Mrs Begum's consultant suggests a trial of ondensetron and steroids, to which she responds dramatically. She is eventually discharged home a week later on oral steroids with a follow-up plan. Her steroid dose is gradually reduced to a maintenance dose by 16 weeks' gestation and eventually stopped at 23 weeks.

The rest of her pregnancy was uneventful and she delivered the twins spontaneously at 37 weeks. The babies had normal Apgar scores and birth weights. She was advised that her symptoms could recur in subsequent pregnancies.

CASE REVIEW

This 29-year-old para 1 presented with vomiting and dehydration in early pregnancy. After excluding the other causes of vomiting the diagnosis was that of HG. The mainstay of management of this condition is rehydration by means of intravenous fluids containing adequate sodium and potassium along with regular antiemetics. HG is associated with increased risk of venous thrombosis, therefore thromboprophylaxis is recommended. Thiamine is prescribed to prevent Wernicke's encephalopathy.

Mrs Begum responded well to conventional treatment; however, she experienced recurrence of her symptoms, which were refractory to hydration and antiemetics. She responded well to ondensetron and corticosteroids, drugs reserved for refractory HG. Corticosteroids were stopped at 23 weeks after a gradual dosage reduction.

The twins born at 37 weeks gestation, were of normal weight and did not require admission to neonatal unit. Thus, with appropriate management there was no evidence of long-term effects of hyperemesis or its treatment for the mother and her babies. In view of her history, Mrs Begum was counselled about the risk of recurrence of symptoms in subsequent pregnancies.

Further reading

Kuscu NK, Koyuncu F. Hyperemesis gravidarum: current concepts and management. *Postgrad Med J* 2002; 78: 76–79.

Neill AM, Nelson-Piercy C. Hyperemesis gravidarum review. *The Obstetrician and Gynaecologist* 2003; 5: 204–207.

A 38-year-old woman with a twin pregnancy

Mrs Akinte is 38-year-old primigravida admitted with severe hyperemesis which has improved with hydration and antiemetics. She has a pelvic ultrasound which confirms a twin pregnancy about which she is delighted as it is a pregnancy following treatment with clomifene citrate for anovulatory primary subfertility.

What are the predisposing factors for twin pregnancy?

These include a family history or previous history of multiple births, increased maternal age, ovulation induction (with clomifene 10%, with gonadotrophins 30% and *in vitro* fertilization [IVF] 25–30%) and race (Japanese 7/1000 pregnancies, Nigerian 40/1000)

KEY POINT

Twins account for about 1% of all pregnancies with two-thirds being dizygotic and one-third monozygotic. The incidence of triplets is 1/4000. There is increased incidence as a consequence of assisted reproductive techniques.

Mrs Akinte wants to know the causes for twin pregnancy and also the different types of twins. What do you tell her?

Twin pregnancy occurs when two or more ova are fertilized to form dizygotic (non-identical) twins, or a single fertilized egg divides to form monozygotic (identical) twins.

In a dizygotic twin pregnancy, each fetus has its own placenta (either separate or fused), amnion and chorion, whereas in a monozygotic pregnancy, the situation is

more complex depending on the timing of the division of the embryo:
• *Embryo splits at 3 days:* two chorions, two amnions (dichorionic, diamniotic)
• *Embryo splits at 4–7 days:* single placenta, one chorion, two amnions (monochorionic, diamniotic)
• *Embryo splits at 8–12 days* (rare): single placenta, one chorion and one amnion (monochorionic, monoamniotic)
• *Embryo splits at 13 days* (very rare): conjoined or Siamese twins

The scan shows the twins to be dichorionic and diamniotic at 10 + 3 weeks' gestation and the heart beat of both the fetuses are seen. Mrs Akinte wishes to know if the twins are identical.

How can you tell if the twins are monozygotic or dizygotic?

While a monochorionic placentation on scan suggests identical (monozygotic twins), with a dichorionic placenta it is not possible to determine zygosity unless the twins are of discordant gender.

Determination of zygosity may be useful for:
• Assisting with medical decisions for the twins in later life (e.g. to establish any genetic risk of illness)
• Participation in twin research studies
• Simply answering the inevitable questions from friends, relatives or strangers

Zygosity can only be conclusively determined by DNA fingerprinting, which requires amniocentesis, chorionic villus sampling (CVS), cordocentesis and after delivery by DNA fingerprinting of cord blood or sending a small swab of cheek cells or a blood sample to the laboratory.

Determination of chorionicity can be performed by ultrasonography and relies on the assessment of fetal gender, number of placentas and characteristics of the membrane between the two amniotic sacs. Different-sex

Obstetrics and Gynaecology: Clinical Cases Uncovered.
By M. Cruickshank and A. Shetty. Published 2009 by Blackwell Publishing. ISBN 978-1-4051-8671-1.

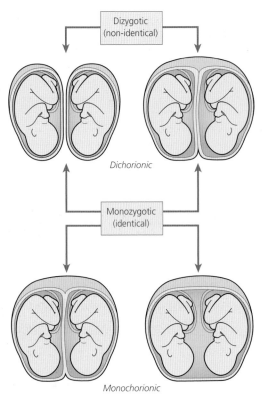

Figure 25.1 Dizygotic and monozygotic twins. In dichorionic twins the inter-twin membrane is composed of a central layer of chorionic tissue sandwiched between two layers of amnion, whereas in monochorionic twins there is no chorionic layer present.

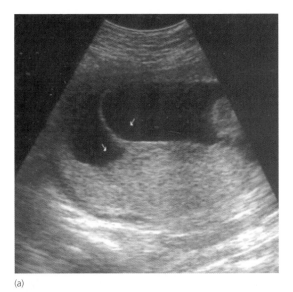

(a)

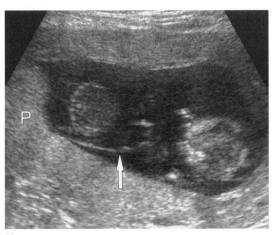

(b)

Figure 25.2 Ultrasound appearance of monochorionic (left) and dichorionic (right) twin pregnancies at around 12 weeks' gestation. The 'lamda' sign is seen in the dichorionic set of twins and the 'T' sign (with the very thin inter-twin membrane) in the monochorionic set of twins.

twins are dizygotic and therefore dichorionic, but in about two-thirds of twin pregnancies the fetuses are of the same sex and these may be either monozygotic or dizygotic (Fig. 25.1). Similarly, if there are two separate placentas the pregnancy is dichorionic.

In dichorionic twins the inter-twin membrane is composed of a central layer of chorionic tissue sandwiched between two layers of amnion, whereas in monochorionic twins there is no chorionic layer present. Dichorionic twins can be easily distinguished by the presence of a thick septum between the chorionic sacs. This septum becomes progressively thinner to form the chorionic component of the inter-twin membrane, but remains thicker and easier to identify at the base of the membrane as a triangular tissue projection, or 'lambda' sign.

Sonographic examination of the base of the inter-twin membrane at 10–14 weeks' gestation for the presence or absence of the lambda sign (Fig. 25.2) provides reliable distinction between dichorionic and monochorionic

pregnancies. With advancing gestation there is regression of the chorion laeve and the 'lambda' sign becomes progressively more difficult to identify.

Mrs Akinte wishes to know the importance of prenatal determination of chorionicity. What information would you give her?

Chorionicity, rather than zygosity, is the main factor determining pregnancy outcome. In monochorionic

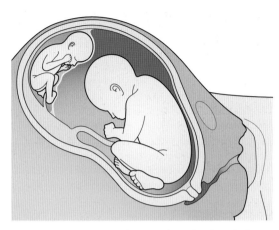

Figure 25.3 Twin–twin transfusion syndrome (TTTS). In the larger recipient there is usually a large bladder and polyhydramnios and the smaller anuric donor is held fixed to the placenta by the collapsed membranes of the anhydramniotic sac.

twins the rates of miscarriage, perinatal death, preterm delivery, fetal growth restriction and fetal abnormalities are much higher than in dichorionic twins. Death of a monochorionic fetus is associated with a high chance of sudden death or severe neurological impairment in the co-twin.

Twin–twin transfusion syndrome (TTTS), an imbalanced flow of blood from one twin to another, occurs in 10–15% of monozygotic twins who share a placenta (Fig. 25.3). The implications of this are very serious for the survival (perinatal mortality of >80%) and health of both twins and they would require close monitoring during the pregnancy.

In view of her age, Mrs Akinte is concerned about the risk of Down's syndrome. What screening investigations would you offer her?

Fetal abnormality is more common in multiple pregnancies – both the maternal age-specific chromosomal disorders (as increasing maternal age is a risk factor for multiple birth) and fetal anatomical disorders (seen more with monochorionic than dichorionic twins).

Serum screening in multiple pregnancy is not reliable, as it may identify only about 45% of affected fetuses for a 5% false positive rate. Nuchal translucency (NT) assessment (ultrasound measurement of the translucency of the nuchal fold in the fetal neck between 10 and 14 weeks) identifies about 70% of individual fetuses at high

risk of trisomy and is an option for screening with multiple pregnancies.

Invasive prenatal diagnosis is challenging as there are at least two fetuses to sample correctly and should be undertaken in a tertiary referral centre. The procedure chosen will depend on chorionicity. Both amniocentesis and CVS risk contamination – amniocentesis where double sac sampling occurs and CVS where chorions are not separately sampled. Procedure-related miscarriage rates appear to be similar to those for singleton pregnancies.

> **KEY POINT**
>
> If one fetus is detected as abnormal, selective termination (if desired) with intracardiac potassium chloride in dichorionic twins must be accurately targeted. Selective termination in monochorionic pregnancies risks co-twin sequelae, but cord occlusion can be considered.

Mrs Akinte opts to have the NT scan at 12 weeks which shows the fetuses to be at low risk for Down's syndrome. She asks about the risks associated with multiple pregnancy.

What do you tell her?

Multiple pregnancies are considered high-risk because:
• Increased risk of prematurity – the mean gestation for twins is 37 weeks and for triplets 31 weeks
• Higher risk of congenital abnormality associated with multiple pregnancies (×2–4 the rate in singleton pregnancies)
• Higher rates of cerebral palsy found in twins (1–1.5%) and triplets (7–8%)
• Perinatal mortality rate for twins is significantly higher than singletons (×5) and even higher for triplets (×6).
• Smaller babies – fetuses tend to be individually smaller than those in a singleton pregnancy because of greater demand for nutrients and slower *in utero* growth, i.e. light-for-dates. Monozygotic twins tend to be smaller than dizygotic twins.
• Death of one fetus. Death of one fetus in dichorionic pregnancies carries a risk of death or handicap of 5–10% to the remaining fetus. This is mainly because of preterm delivery, which may be the consequence of release of cytokines and prostaglandins by the resorbing dead placenta. In monochorionic twins, there is at least a 30% risk of death or neurological handicap to the co-twin because, in addition to preterm delivery, there is a risk of

---

> **Box 25.1 Complications specific to monochorionic twin pregnancy**
>
> *Twin–twin transfusion syndrome (TTTS)* with placental vascular anastomosis with unequal distribution of blood between the twins. Approximately 10–15% of monochorionic twin pregnancies may be affected with TTTS. The donor twin becomes anaemic, hypovolaemic, oligohydramniotic and growth restricted. The recipient becomes polycythaemic, hypovolaemic and polyuric with polyhydramniosis and hydrops.
>
> *Twin reversed arterial perfusion sequence (TRAP)* is found in approximately 1% of monozygotic twin pregnancies (acardiac twinning). The underlying mechanism is thought to be disruption of normal vascular perfusion and development of the recipient twin because of an umbilical arterial–arterial anastomosis with the donor or pump-twin.

> **Box 25.2 Management of twin pregnancies**
>
> Monochorionic twins should be scanned fortnightly from 16 weeks to detect twin–twin transfusion syndrome (TTTS). The pathognomonic features of severe TTTS by ultrasonographic examination are the presence of a large bladder in the polyuric recipient fetus in the polyhydramniotic sac and 'absent' bladder in the anuric donor which is much smaller than the recipient (Fig. 25.2). If suspected, these pregnancies should be referred to tertiary fetal medicine centres for further management – first line management is usually laser surgery of inter-twin vascular placental anastomoses where the syndrome develops before 26 weeks' gestation, other options include serial amnioreduction or elective delivery.

acute hypotensive episodes as a result of haemorrhage from the live fetus into the dead fetoplacental unit (Box 25.1).
• Higher rate of maternal pregnancy-related complications such as hyperemesis gravidarum, miscarriage, polyhydramnios, pre-eclampsia, anaemia and antepartum haemorrhage.
• Higher rate of complications in labour – malpresentation, vasa praevia, cord prolapse, premature separation of placenta, cord entanglement and postpartum haemorrhage (PPH).

Mrs Akinte wants some information on support groups. What support groups do you know of?
• TAMBA: Twin and multiple birth association
• The Multiple Birth Foundation
• The UK Twin to Twin Transfusion Syndrome Association

What kind of antenatal care can she expect during this twin pregnancy?
• Detailed anomaly scan at 18–20 weeks.
• Cervical length scan at 20–24 weeks to determine the risk of preterm labour. Cervical length <2.5 mm is associated with increased risk of preterm labour, hence prophylactic steroids could be offered. There is not enough evidence about the role of cervical cerclage, but this too could be offered.

• Regular scans every 4 weeks after about 24 weeks until 32 weeks, to monitor growth and fetal well-being, thereafter 2-weekly until 36 weeks. From 36 week onwards umbilical artery Doppler scan and amniotic fluid volume should be performed weekly (Box 25.2).
• Anaemia should be looked for and treated vigorously.
• Monitor for early signs of pre-eclampsia.

Her 20-week detailed anomaly scan was normal. The 24-week scan showed normal growth of both the twins with normal liquor volume. The cervical length was found to be 41 mm which is within normal limits. Her husband works offshore.

She is keen to know her likelihood of having a full-term pregnancy and how big the babies are likely to be when born?
See Table 25.1.

Table 25.1 Gestation periods for multiple births.

	Average length of pregnancy (weeks)	Average birth weight (kg)
Singletons	40	3.5
Twins	37	2.5
Triplets	34	1.8
Quads	32	1.4

Mrs Akinte is seen at the clinic at 28 weeks, and the growth scan shows the abdominal circumference of both the fetuses to be on the 50th centile with normal liquor volumes. Twin 1, which is the leading twin, was transverse and twin 2 was breech. Mrs Akinte is anxious about the presentation of the fetus and having a caesarean section.

How would you counsel her?

As Mrs Akinte is only 28 weeks at present, it is highly likely that the lie and presentation might change as the pregnancy advances. She could attempt a trial of vaginal delivery provided the first twin is a cephalic presentation and there are no other complicating factors. Where the first twin is presenting as breech or as a transverse lie, caesarean section is the preferred mode of delivery.

Her 32- and 34-week scans show normal growth and normal liquor of both the twins. At 36 weeks abdominal circumference of twin 1 is on 50th centile but twin 2's abdominal circumference is just above 10th centile. The liquor volume of both the twins is normal and there is good end diastolic flow on the umbilical artery Doppler scan. The presentation of twin 1 is cephalic and that of twin 2 breech.

How would you manage her?

Repeat umbilical artery Doppler scan in a week's time at 37 weeks.

Mrs Akinte feels good fetal movements for both twins. On scan twin 1's abdominal circumference is still on 50th centile but twin 2's abdominal circumference is now on the 5th centile with static growth. Twin 1 is still cephalic and twin 2 is breech.

What would you advise her?

Admission to the ward for induction of labour because of static growth of twin 2. If the cervix is unfavourable, prostaglandins would be indicated for induction of labour, if favourable, artificial rupture of membranes (ARM) with oxytocin augmentation could be performed.

Consider induction of labour for pregnancy complications. It is uncommon for twin pregnancies to be allowed to progress beyond 40 completed weeks. There are insufficient data available to support a practice of elective delivery from 37 weeks' gestation for women with an otherwise uncomplicated twin pregnancy at term although the general practice is to deliver by 37–39 weeks.

Mrs Akinte's cervix is 3 cm dilated and favorable. She has an ARM and oxytocin is commenced. Both the fetuses are monitored continuously by cardiotocography (CTG). She wishes to have an early epidural for pain relief which is organized.

What would be your intrapartum management?

Obtain IV access, FBC, group and save, monitor fetal heart rates separately and check position of lead fetus.

In most cases, vaginal birth proceeds as normal. Immediately after first baby is born determine the position of the second fetus by abdominal and vaginal examination with or without ultrasound. Rupture the second amniotic sac (once the presenting part is fixed in the pelvis) and proceed to delivery (as either breech or cephalic).

If transverse, external cephalic or internal podalic version can be attempted to bring the baby into a longitudinal lie. A caesarean section for the second twin may be indicated if version is unsuccessful or if there is fetal distress.

Oxytocin augmentation of uterine contractions may be required after delivery of twin 1. The second twin usually delivers within 20–45 minutes of the first twin, although this can vary.

The question of whether all women with twin pregnancies should have a caesarean section is contentious. Current NICE guidance recognizes that in uncomplicated twin pregnancies at term with a cephalic first twin, the second twin nonetheless has a higher risk of perinatal morbidity and mortality – whether section for the second twin improves outcome is uncertain and therefore should not be routinely offered, except as part of research.

Third stage should be actively managed by IM injection of syntometrine or syntocinon to avoid PPH.

> **KEY POINT**
>
> Monochorionic, monoamniotic placentation is found in approximately 1% of all twin gestations. High mortality rates (up to 50%) have been attributed to cord entanglement, knots and twists, congenital anomalies and prematurity.

Mrs Akinte progresses normally in the first and second stage of labour. Both the fetal heart traces remain reassuring throughout labour. Following the delivery of the first twin, the second twin is confirmed to be in a transverse lie. External cephalic version is performed and once the head is stabilized in the pelvis, an ARM is performed. There is good descent of the fetal head with contractions, but because of fetal

bradycardia, a ventouse delivery is performed uneventfully. The third stage is managed actively with syntometrine and syntocinon infusion. The placenta with the membranes is delivered complete. The uterus is well contracted and the total blood loss is 700 mL. The babies are in good condition and do not need admission to neonatal unit.

CASE REVIEW

Mrs Akinte had an early diagnosis of a dichorionic twin pregnancy at 10 weeks' gestation. She opted to have nuchal scans on the twins which gave both the twins a low risk for Down's syndrome. She was given information about the support groups, risks of twin pregnancy, antenatal management and intrapartum care plans. The detailed scan, booking bloods and all the growth scans up until 34 weeks were normal. Twin 2's growth began to tail off towards 36 weeks and was static by 37 weeks, and delivery was planned. As twin 1 was in a cephalic presentation, Mrs Akinte opted for a vaginal delivery. Labour was induced with an ARM and oxytocin and progressed normally and she delivered both babies vaginally. The third stage was managed actively with acceptable blood loss of 700 mL.

KEY POINTS

- When a multiple gestation has been diagnosed every effort should be made to determine chorionicity at the time of diagnosis. The optimal time to determine chorionicity is 10–14 weeks
- Biochemical screening for aneuploidy is not recommended in twins. NT screening is useful for identifying twin pregnancies at high risk of aneuploidy
- Invasive prenatal diagnosis is technically more demanding in multiple pregnancies than singleton pregnancies
- Routine hospitalization for bed rest in multiple gestation is *not* recommended. There is insufficient evidence to support prophylactic activity restriction or work leave in multiple gestation
- An 18–22 week detailed anomaly scan is advised
- Serial ultrasonographic evaluation every 4 weeks is indicated in dichorionic twin gestations to confirm

  normal growth and fortnightly in uncomplicated monochorionic twin pregnancy to look for features suggestive of TTTS and to monitor growth
- Multiple pregnancies are associated with increased risks of antenatal complications such as miscarriage, preterm birth, intrauterine growth restriction, anaemia, pre-eclampsia, antepartum haemorrhage and gestational diabetes
- For otherwise uncomplicated twin pregnancies, delivery should be considered at 38–39 weeks
- Vaginal delivery is an appropriate mode of delivery for uncomplicated twin pregnancies with the first twin in vertex presentation. The clinical indications for elective caesarean section in twin gestations include a non-vertex first twin and monoamniotic twins

Case 26 A 26-year-old woman diagnosed HIV positive on routine antenatal screening

Mrs Oktie-ebuh, a 26-year-old, attends her local surgery requesting antenatal care. She has recently moved to the UK from Nigeria to join her husband who is a student at the local university. She is 16 weeks' pregnant and had her initial care in Nigeria, including a dating scan. Her community midwife carries out the antenatal check up and provides her with information about the care in her pregnancy. She also obtains blood for routine antenatal screening including an infection screen after consent.

Ten days later, Mrs Oktie-ebuh receives a letter from the obstetric consultant with a clinic appointment to discuss the results of her recent blood tests. Her blood results are as below:

Hb	*135 g/L*
Blood group	*O rhesus positive*
Down's syndrome screening risk	*1 : 1856*
Serum alpha-fetaprotein	*<2 Mean of median*
Rubella screen	*Immune*
Treponema pallidum	*Negative*
HIV screen	*Positive*
Hepatitis B screen	*Hepatitis B surface Antigen: positive*
	Hepatitis B core Antigen: negative
	Hepatitis B core Antibody: positive
	Hepatitis e Antigen: negative

Mrs Oktie-ebuh wonders what could be the problem with the blood tests, as she feels well and, so far, has had an uneventful pregnancy.

Obstetrics and Gynaecology: Clinical Cases Uncovered.
By M. Cruickshank and A. Shetty. Published 2009 by Blackwell Publishing. ISBN 978-1-4051-8671-1.

How will you interpret these blood results?

Her results indicate that she is rhesus positive and not anaemic. She is at low risk for having a baby with Down's syndrome and spina bifida. She has tested positive for HIV infection and has chronic hepatitis B infection.

KEY POINT

Pregnant women should be offered screening for HIV early in pregnancy as appropriate interventions can reduce maternal–child transmission.

What important issues will you consider when counselling this woman who has tested positive for HIV infection?

This diagnosis may be profoundly shocking and a life-changing experience for the woman and therefore needs sensitive handling. As a clinician some important issues to consider are:
• Confidentiality
• Empathy while communicating the results
• HIV status of partner
• HIV status of existing children

What specific information do you need from Mrs Oktie-ebuh's history and examination?

• Details of any medical problems including medications and the pregnancy so far
• Past obstetric history:
  ○ previous pregnancies

Box 26.1 HIV: burden of infection

Approximately 3 million HIV positive pregnant women give birth each year, of whom 75% reside in sub-Saharan Africa, which also accounts for most of the 700,000 new HIV infections among children annually

Prevalence of HIV among pregnant women is on the rise in the UK, especially in the inner city areas of London, and most of these women are of black African ethnicity.

In 2005, 1100 children were born to HIV positive women in the UK.

Box 26.2 Psychosocial issues

- HIV positive pregnant women should be encouraged to disclose their HIV status to their partner
- Testing of any existing children for HIV is recommended
- A thorough early assessment of social circumstances of a newly diagnosed HIV positive pregnant woman is essential

---

　　○　gestation at delivery
　　○　mode of delivery
- Past history of blood transfusion and sexually transmitted infections
- Patient's awareness of her HIV and hepatitis status
- HIV status of her existing children and partner
- Assessment of her social circumstances (Box 26.2)
- Detailed general and systemic examination

Mrs Oktie-ebuh is a primigravida who has had an uneventful pregnancy so far. She is fit and well and denies any major medical problems, including any allergies. There are no abnormalities noted on examination.

She was unaware of her HIV and hepatitis status and is upset and shocked at disclosure of the test results. During the long consultation, her consultant explained in detail the implications of her HIV and hepatitis status, including the effect of the diagnosis on her pregnancy. She also discussed the measures for combating the risk of transmission to her baby and the need for compliance with clinic appointments and the recommended treatment, which would be overseen by a specialist team of medical personnel experienced in dealing with HIV infections (Boxes 26.3 & 26.4).

Box 26.3 HIV in pregnancy

- Mother–child transmission of HIV varies between 15% and 30% in untreated or undiagnosed mothers
- In absence of intervention, >80% of perinatal transmissions occur late in the third trimester, intrapartum (majority) and postnatally through breastfeeding
- Vertical transmission can be reduced to <1% with appropriate measures
- Interventions include:
- antiretroviral therapy (ART) to mother and neonate
- prelabour caesarean section (PLCS)
- avoidance of breastfeeding
- Advanced maternal disease, low CD4 lymphocyte counts and high plasma viral load are associated with an increased risk of transmission
- Principal obstetric risk factors for transmission are vaginal delivery in the presence of a significant viral load, duration of membrane rupture and delivery prior to 32 completed weeks' gestation
- Pregnancy does not adversely affect HIV progression or survival
- Earlier studies had suggested an association between HIV and an increased risk of miscarriage, preterm delivery and intrauterine growth restriction but more recent studies have not confirmed this
- With advances in ART, HIV infection in the industrialized world is regarded as a carrier state or chronic infection
- Symptomatic disease is rare and can be associated with opportunistic infections (e.g. *Pneumocystis*, cytomegalovirus, *Toxoplasma*)

Box 26.4 HIV and hepatitis B virus co-infection

- Materno-fetal transmission of hepatitis B virus (HBV) infection is related to the level of viraemia
- Transmission is >90% in women positive for HbeAg compared to 40% transmission in women negative for HbeAg
- Active measures can effectively prevent transmission to fetus. These measures include hepatitis B vaccination of the infants born to HBsAg positive mothers at birth, 1 month, 2 months and 12 months of age. In infants born to mothers with high risk of infectivity (HBeAg positive), HBV immunoglobulin at birth is also indicated
- Pregnant women with HIV–HBV co-infection should be treated with a regimen that includes agents active against HIV and HBV as required

What other investigations would you like to carry out at this stage?

Obtain blood for:

- Plasma viral load
- CD4 lymphocyte count
- HIV genotype
- Hepatitis C screen
- Full blood count, baseline liver function and renal function tests
- Haemoglobinopathy screen in view of her ethnicity

KEY POINT

Maternal plasma viral load is the *strongest* predictor of vertical transmission. Low or undetectable plasma viral load is associated with very low risk of transmission.

Screening for genital infections

Infections to be screened for include: *Chlamydia trachomatis*, *Nisseria gonorrhoea*, *Bacterial vaginosis* and *Treponema pallidum* serology. Screening should be carried out at presentation and repeated in the third trimester. Any infection should be treated as per national guidelines including a test for cure and partner notification as indicated to prevent reinfection.

KEY POINT

There is a higher prevalence of sexually transmitted infection amongst HIV positive women. Evidence suggests that the risk of chorioamnionitis, premature rupture of membranes (PROM) and preterm labour increased in presence of genital infections. Antenatal HIV care should be delivered by a multidisciplinary team consisting of HIV physician, obstetrician, paediatrician and specialist midwife along with involvement of the woman's GP, community midwife, social workers and voluntary support groups as required.

The results of Mrs Oktie-ebuh's investigations are as follows:

Hb	133 g/L
Haemoglobinopathy screen	No haemoglobinpathy detected
Renal and liver function tests	Within normal limits
Hepatitis C screen	Negative
Plasma viral load for HIV	14,000 copies/mL
CD4 lymphocyte count	340×10^6/L
HIV genotype	HIV 1, non-B subtype (subtype A) (Box 26.5)
Genital infection screen	Negative

Box 26.5 HIV types: HIV 1 and HIV 2

- Most HIV infections in Europe are with HIV type 1
- Infection with HIV type 2 is usually limited to West Africa; however, with global migration the population dynamics are changing
- Although the two are related, there are important differences between HIV 1 and HIV 2 that influence natural history, pathogenicity and response to therapy
- Making the correct diagnosis is important as therapy differs significantly if HIV 2 is detected
- NNRTIs of ART have no activity against HIV 2

Not all laboratories differentiate between the two virus types, so it is important that patients at risk of HIV 2 have appropriate investigations performed

---

How will you manage this woman who has been diagnosed with HIV infection at 18 weeks' gestation?

The aim of management is to minimize the risk of materno-fetal transmission while not increasing maternal or neonatal morbidity.

Specific management

- Antiretroviral therapy
- Obstetric management

Mr and Mrs Oktie-ebuh attended the combined multidisciplinary clinic as arranged. Mr Oktie-ebuh had his blood taken for HIV screening.

The HIV physician discussed the treatment options and explained that in view of the high viral load she would require a combination of three antiretroviral drugs to minimize the risk of materno-fetal transmission. The effect of therapy would be monitored regularly with viral load estimation by means of blood tests.

The couple's main concern was the effect of the antiviral therapy on the pregnancy and their baby.

What are the side-effects of antiretroviral therapy?
Antiretroviral therapy

Of more than 20 compounds currently licensed for treatment of HIV 1 infections in the UK, only ziduvidine (ZDV) is specifically indicated for use in pregnancy. Information about safety of antiretroviral therapy (ART) in pregnancy is limited. The risk of transmission should

Table 26.1 Classes of drugs used for antiretroviral therapy in pregnancy along with their side-effects.

Classification	Examples	Problems
Nucleoside reverse transcriptase inhibitor (NRTI)	Ziduvidine (ZDV)	Well tolerated
	Lamivudine	Lactic acidosis (rare)
	Stavudine	Hepatic dysfunction
Protease inhibitor (PI)	Indinavir	Gastrointestinal side-effects (common)
	Saquinavir	Anaemia
		Hepatic dysfunction
Non-nucleoside reverse transcriptase inhibitor (NNRTI)	Nevirapine	Hepatic toxicity
		Rash, Stevens–Johnson syndrome

be balanced against the toxicities of ART. Apart from didanosine and efavirenz, embryonal toxicity has not been reported with other drugs (Table 26.1).

Treatment regimens

Efficacy relates to reducing infection in the neonate, maintaining or improving maternal health and preserving maternal therapeutic options.

Ziduvidine monotherapy

ZDV monotherapy is a valid option for women:
• With a viral load <6–10,000 HIV RNA copies/mL
• Not requiring combination therapy for their own health
• Not wishing to take combination therapy
• Willing to deliver by prelabour caaesarean section (PLCS)
• To commence prior to 30 weeks
  ZDV in combination with PLCS is said to reduce the risk of transmission to <1%.

Highly active antiretroviral therapy

Highly active antiretroviral therapy (HAART) is a combination therapy containing three or more drugs and usually includes two nucleoside reverse transcriptase inhibitors (NRTIs) plus non-nucleoside reverse transcriptase inhibitor (NNRTI)/boosted protease inhibitor (PI). The indications for the use of HAART in pregnancy are:

> **Box 26.6 Monitoring antiretroviral therapy**
>
> ART is monitored using HIV plasma viral load, CD4 lymphocyte count and clinical status. Plasma viral load is the most important determinant of mother–child transmission
>   Viral load should be quantified:
> • At presentation
> • At least every 3 months and at 36 weeks in women on established therapy
> • Two weeks after starting or changing therapy
> • At delivery
>
>   *A second assay should be used where there are discrepancies between the viral load, CD4 cell count and the clinical status*

• For maternal health
• If baseline viral load >10,000 HIV RNA copies/mL and no maternal indication for HAART, commencing at 22–24 weeks
• As an alternative to ZDV monotherapy and PLCS
• Drug resistance detected on genotype or phenotype
• Therapy commenced prior to pregnancy should be continued throughout pregnancy
  Evidence suggests that use of HAART is associated with preterm delivery, especially before 34 weeks.

Short-term antiretroviral therapy

Short-term antiretroviral therapy (START) is HAART used for prevention of mother–child transmission during pregnancy. It should be discontinued after delivery when viral load <50 copies/mL.

It was discussed with the couple that although there were limited safety data on the effects of ART in pregnancy, evidence suggests that in general it is well tolerated and appears reasonably safe for the mother and the baby (Box 26.6).

Obstetric management of pregnancy and delivery
Antenatal care

The important aspects of antenatal care are confidentiality, multidisciplinary approach and instituting an agreed care plan. Periconceptual folic acid (5 mg/day) is recommended, especially if the woman is on co-trimoxazole for *Pneumocystis* prophylaxis. Dating scan, serum screening and mid-trimester anomaly scan should be offered routinely.

During her pregnancy Mrs Oktie-ebuh is reviewed regularly at the multidisciplinary clinic. She has tolerated the three drug HAART regimen very well with no evidence of any side-effects. The plasma HIV RNA viral load showed a dramatic response to the ART and was <50 copies/mL (undetectable) at 30 weeks' gestation.

Her pregnancy is progressing well. Infection screen for genital infections is repeated at 28 weeks and reported as negative. She is now 34 weeks' pregnant and is due to attend the clinic to discuss a plan for her delivery.

What are the important factors to consider when deciding the mode of delivery for a HIV positive pregnant woman? How will you help this woman to make an informed choice?

Vaginal delivery would be an option for Mrs Oktie-ebuh as her viral load was <50 copies/mL. Precautions to minimize the risk of transmission – including *avoiding* an early artificial rupture of membranes (ARM), fetal blood sampling (if there were concerns about fetal well-being) and a fetal scalp electrode in labour – would be advised (Box 26.7).

KEY POINT

Prelabour caesarean section has been shown to reduce the risk of perinatal HIV transmission and is of most benefit in women with a high viral load.

Mrs Oktie-ebuh opted for a PLCS, which was arranged for 39 weeks. She was advised to seek help if she laboured prior to the arranged procedure.

Postnatal care

Breastfeeding constitutes a transmission risk despite ART and is therefore *not* recommended. Consider cabergoline for lactation suppression if indicated. Watch for postnatal depression as women of this group are at increased risk of depression post delivery.

Care of the neonate

All babies born to HIV positive mothers should be followed up by a paediatrician. Infants should be given ZDV or alternative suitable monotherapy for 4 weeks. Triple therapy should be given to neonates born to untreated mothers or women with detectable viraemia despite combination therapy.

Mrs Oktie-ebuh underwent an uneventful caesarean section as scheduled. She delivered a baby boy weighing 3.78 kg in good condition with normal Apgar scores. The baby was exclusively formula fed as per plan. All relevant investigations were carried out for screening and the baby was commenced on oral AZT. He also received a vaccination against hepatitis B.

The mother and baby made an uneventful recovery and were discharged home 7 days after the procedure. Arrangements were made to follow the baby at the paediatric clinic, while Mrs Oktie-ebuh was to be reviewed at the clinic by her HIV physician.

Contraceptive advice was given supplemented by leaflets prior to her discharge from the hospital.

Box 26.7 Mode and timing of delivery

A blanket policy of caesarean section for all HIV positive women is not appropriate, but HIV should be taken into equation when considering mode of delivery for obstetric, medical and patient preference indications.

In addition to obstetric indications, PLCS is indicated for:
• Women on ZDV monotherapy
• Women on combination therapy with detectable viraemia

PLCS should be considered for women with HIV–HCV co-infection. PLCS should be planned for:
• 38 weeks if on ZDV monotherapy or with detectable viraemia
• 39 weeks if on HAART and undetectable viraemia

Vaginal delivery is an option for women with undetectable viraemia on HAART. If anticipating a vaginal delivery avoid induction of labour, leave the membranes intact for as long as possible and avoid invasive fetal monitoring and traumatic instrumental delivery.

Intravenous ZDV is indicated predelivery for mothers on ZDV monotherapy or >50 HIV RNA copies/mL on HAART.

CASE REVIEW

This 26-year-old well Nigerian woman booked at 16 weeks' gestation at her local GP surgery for antenatal care in her first pregnancy. The results of the routine screening blood tests indicated that she was HIV positive and was a carrier for hepatitis B virus infection. The importance of offering antenatal screening for infections should not be underestimated as appropriate diagnosis and timely interventions can minimize the risk of vertical transmission of infections. This woman was a recent migrant from a high-risk area and was therefore at increased risk of such an infection. There is a higher prevalence of other sexually transmitted infections amongst this group of women, as was the case with this woman, who was found to be a carrier for hepatitis B virus infection. The sexually transmitted infection screen is an important aspect of management as these infections can lead to an increased incidence of PROM and preterm labour, possibly as a result of chorioamnionitis.

This woman was appropriately managed in a multidisciplinary setting and was commenced on a three drug ART (HAART) regimen for prevention of vertical transmission at 18 weeks. Combination therapy is indicated in women with HIV viral load >10,000 HIV RNA copies/mL even if the ART is not for maternal health reasons. If the viral load is <6–10,000 copies/mL and the patient is willing to deliver by a PLCS, then ZDV monotherapy is an option. If ART is not indicated for maternal health, it is commenced late in second trimester to minimize the adverse effects.

Maternal viral load is the most important determinant of the risk of vertical transmission. Although the safety data for ART use in pregnancy are not extensive, apart from didanosine and efavirenz there have been no concerns raised about embryo toxicity. This patient tolerated the ART well and her plasma viral load showed a dramatic decline to <50 copies/mL over few weeks, indicating a good response.

The mode of delivery was discussed at 34 weeks' gestation and the advantages and disadvantages of a caesarean delivery and vaginal birth were also discussed along with supporting evidence. Until recently, a PLCS was thought to be the optimum mode of delivery for pregnant women with HIV infection. However, more recent evidence suggests that in women with undetectable viral load on HAART, there is an option of a vaginal delivery as the risk of vertical transmission is minimal.

This woman opted for a PLCS, which was performed at 39 weeks. Her baby was tested for HIV infection and commenced on ZDV monotherapy prophylaxis to further prevent the risk of infection. He also received vaccination against hepatitis B virus infection to prevent transmission of infection.

Breastfeeding is an important means of HIV transmission and is contraindicated to help minimize the risk.

Adequate follow-up was arranged for both the mother and her baby with the HIV physicians and paediatricians, respectively. She was also given contraceptive advice prior to her discharge from the hospital.

KEY POINTS

- Prevalence of HIV infection among pregnant women is on the rise in the UK
- Antenatal screening for HIV should be offered to all pregnant women early in pregnancy
- HIV positive pregnant women should be screened for genital infections at pregnancy and at 28 weeks
- Interventions such as ART, delivery by PLCS and avoidance of breastfeeding reduces the transmission risk from 15–20% to <1%
- Pregnant women with HIV infection are best managed by a multidisciplinary team
- Safety data on the use of ART in pregnancy are limited
- Maternal plasma viral load is the most important determinant of mother–child transmission
- Mode of delivery should be discussed around 34–36 weeks and should involve the women, her obstetrician and the HIV physician
- Vaginal delivery is an option for women with undetectable viraemia on HAART
- All babies born to HIV positive mothers should be followed up by a paediatrician and receive appropriate ART

Further reading

British HIV and Children's HIV guidelines on the management of HIV infection in pregnant women. *HIV Medicine* 2008; 9: 452–502.

Royal College of Paediatrics and Child Health. *Reducing mother to child transmission of HIV. Update Report of an Intercollegiate Working Party Report.* July 2006.

MCQs

For each situation, choose the single option you feel is most correct.

a. Progestogen only implant is not as effective as the COC as it does not inhibit ovulation

b. Bleeding will be predictable, unlike the COC

c. The risk of deep venous thrombosis is decreased in COC users

d. The progestogen only implant protects against sexually transmitted infections (STIs)

e. A common reason for discontinuing progestogen only methods is unpredictable bleeding

Which of the following statements is the single best answer?

a. A menstrual history will not be useful in the assessment of this patient

b. A serum follicle stimulating hormone (FSH) level of 70 IU/L is diagnostic of the menopause

c. Herbal remedies can safely be used alongside prescribed medication

d. Oestrogen levels consistently <0.11 mmol/L indicate ovarian failure

e. Combined hormone replacement therapy (HRT) consists of two different oestrogens

Which of the following statements is the single best answer?

a. Your consultation should include review of her respiratory symptoms and smoking

b. A Cusco's speculum should be used for vaginal examination

c. Pelvic floor exercises should be performed on a weekly basis

d. Surgical management should be considered as first line treatment

e. A ring pessary is unlikely to be useful for this patient because of her comorbidity

a. Stratification of the squamous epithelium results from maturation and differentiation

b. The squamo-columnar junction is sited at the external cervical os

c. Squamous metaplasia results from human papillomavirus (HPV) infection

d. A normal cervical appearance on examination excludes a *Chlamydia* infection

e. Cervical ectopy usually requires treatment with cryotherapy

Obstetrics and Gynaecology: Clinical Cases Uncovered.
By M. Cruickshank and A. Shetty. Published 2009 by Blackwell Publishing. ISBN 978-1-4051-8671-1.

5 *A 28-year-old nulliparous woman is referred to colposcopy with a moderately dyskaryotic smear.*

Which of the following statements is the single best answer?

a. Sixty per cent of women with moderate dyskaryosis will have abnormal vaginal bleeding
b. Referral was inappropriate as she has a low risk of having high grade cervical intraepithelial neoplasia (CIN)
c. A diagnostic biopsy must be taken before treatment with cold coagulation
d. Most women require a general anaesthetic for the treatment of CIN
e. She should be offered HPV vaccination to treat her abnormal smear

6 *A 54-year-old woman presents with postmenopausal bleeding after the menopause at age 50. She had a right-sided mastectomy and lymph node sampling 2 years previously for breast cancer and is currently on tamoxifen.*

Which of the following statements is the single best answer?

a. Tamoxifen is an oestrogen antagonist and reduces the risk of endometrial cancer
b. Thickened endometrium with cystic spaces on TV scan suggests endometrial cancer
c. She should have a speculum examination to identify any cervical pathology
d. She should be investigated by an outpatient endometrial biopsy
e. The mostly likely cause of her symptoms is metastatic breast cancer

7 *A 75-year-old woman presents with a 10-year history of vulval itch and irritation. This has failed to respond to avoiding irritants and topical emollients. On examination, the skin is thickened and white round the introitus and perianal skin with superficial ulceration at the fourchette.*

Which is the single most likely cause of her symptoms?

a. Vulval vestibulitis
b. Vulvovaginal thrush
c. Bartholin's abscess
d. Lichen sclerosus
e. Genital warts

8 *A 33-year-old para 2 is admitted as an emergency with rapid onset of acute right iliac fossa pain. On admission, she has tenderness and guarding in her right iliac fossa. Her temperature is 37.8 °C, her pulse is 92 beats/minute and her blood pressure 115/75 mmHg, her white cell count and neutrophil count are both raised.*

Which of the following is the single most likely diagnosis?

a. Endometriosis
b. Torsion of an ovarian cyst
c. Threatened miscarriage
d. Unruptured ectopic pregnancy
e. Mittelschmerz

9 *In the investigation of a 32-year-old para 2 an incidental finding of a pelvic mass is made.*

Which of the following statements is the single best answer?

a. Pregnancy needs to be excluded
b. CT scan is the imaging method of choice
c. Ovarian cancer is the most likely diagnosis
d. Premenopausal status increases her risk of the mass being malignant
e. The diagnosis is unlikely to be fibroids as she is asymptomatic

10 *A 36-year-old woman complains of vaginal discharge and a high vaginal swab shows bacterial vaginosis.*

Which of the following statements is the single best answer?

a. This is caused by a *Trichomonas vaginalis* infection
b. This is a sexually transmitted infection
c. This may have been caused by her intrauterine device
d. She may have noticed a fishy smell
e. Her partner should be treated with penicillin

11 *A 23-year-old woman presents to her GP with rapid onset of severe vulval pain. On examination, her vulva is very swollen and tender.*

Which of the following statements is the single best answer?
a. A full sexual history should be taken initially to make a diagnosis
b. Examination is not essential as a good history and self-sampling will lead to the diagnosis
c. A tender fluctuant swelling over the mons pubis suggests a Bartholin's abscess
d. A herpes infection may be complicated by acute urinary retention
e. A skin biopsy may be required to make the diagnosis

12 *An 18-year-old girl presents with a 3-month history of recurrent postcoital bleeding. She denies any recent sexual activity.*

Which of the following statements is the single best answer?
a. In view of her history, she does not need a *Chlamydia* test
b. She should be offered a cervical screening test
c. You should ask about her current method of contraception and its usage
d. You do not need to offer her a chaperone if the doctor is female
e. She should be referred for colposcopy

13 *In the management of a woman with dysfunctional uterine bleeding.*

Which of the following statements is the single best answer?
a. Mirena intrauterine system (IUS) is a recognized treatment
b. An endometrial biopsy is not usually recommended in a woman aged 45 years
c. Hysterectomy is often recommended as first line therapy
d. Following endometrial ablation, women can discontinue their contraception
e. Gonadotrophin releasing hormone (GnRH) analogues can be used for long-term management

14 *A 32-year-old woman is being investigated for primary infertility. She has not used any contraception for the last 18 months and her normal menstrual cycle is $\kappa = 5–7/35$.*

Which of the following statements is the single best answer?
a. The prevalence of infertility in the UK population is 1 in 17
b. You should check her serum progesterone on day 14 to detect ovulation
c. You need to check her serum testosterone level because of her cycle length
d. Her rubella immunity should be checked
e. First line investigations include laparoscopy and dye test to check tubal patency

15 *Her partner is aged 35 and has no previous children or significant past medical history.*

Which of the following statements is the single best answer?
a. A semen analysis should be performed only if his partner's infertility investigations are normal
b. The normal reference range for minimum sperm count with ejaculate is >30,000,000
c. The presence of small testicular size and azoospermia is suggestive of an obstructive cause
d. The finding of azoospermia suggests that you should arrange to repeat his semen analysis
e. The finding of azoospermia suggests that you should perform a cystic fibrosis screen

16 *A 37-year-old para 2 who is 36 weeks pregnant presents to the day assessment ward with fresh bleeding per vaginum.*

What feature on history and examination would make placenta praevia an unlikely diagnosis?
a. Transverse lie of the fetus
b. A tender hypertonic uterus
c. Her first two deliveries having been by caesarean section
d. Stable maternal condition
e. Good fetal movements, stable fetal condition (e.g. normal fetal heart)

17 *A 24-year-old para 0 is 29 weeks pregnant and presents with leaking clear fluid per vaginum. Her uterus is soft and she is not in labour. The baby is in a cephalic position with the head four-fifths palpable per abdomen, and the fetal heart is regular. Preterm prelabour rupture of membranes is diagnosed.*

What would you not do?
a. Perform a vaginal swab
b. Administer a course of steroids for fetal lung maturity
c. Take bloods for full blood count (including white cell count) and C-reactive protein
d. Start antibiotics (erythromycin)
e. Induce labour as soon as possible

18 *Which of these is not a risk factor for atonic postpartum haemorrhage?*

a. A long labour with oxytocin augmentation
b. High parity
c. Multiple pregnancy
d. Epidural for pain relief
e. Placental abruption

19 *Which of these is not a symptom or sign of impending eclampsia?*

a. Headaches
b. Epigastric pain
c. Frequency of micturition
d. Blurring of vision
e. Hyper-reflexia

20 *Which of these is a routinely offered antenatal screening test in the UK?*

a. Chorionic villus sampling
b. Amniocentesis
c. Screening for HBV infection
d. Screening for group B streptococcus
e. Screening for toxoplasmosis

21 *Which of these is not a risk factor for venous thrombosis?*

a. Hyperemesis gravidarum
b. Malposition of the fetus
c. Smoking
d. Postpartum haemorrhage
e. Puerperal sepsis
f. Increasing maternal age

22 *Which of the following is a relative contraindication for an external cephalic version?*

a. Previous caesarean section
b. Multiparity
c. Extended breech presentation
d. >38 weeks' gestation
e. Maternal shoe size 3

23 *Which of these are not a sign of scar rupture or dehiscence with a vaginal birth after caesarean section (VBAC)?*

a. Fresh bleeding per vaginum
b. Tense and hypertonic uterus
c. Scar tenderness
d. Maternal tachycardia
e. Fetal heart deceleration

24 *Components of the cervical Bishop's score.*

Which is the odd one out?
a. Station of the fetal head
b. Position of the fetal head
c. Cervical dilatation
d. Length of the cervix
e. Consistency of the cervix

25 *Which of the following is a complication of pre-eclampsia?*

a. Fetal macrosomia
b. Pulmonary odema
c. Prelabour preterm rupture of membranes
d. Polyhydramnios
e. Fetal malposition

26 *Which of these statements about twin pregnancies is not true?*

a. All dichorionic pregnancies are dizygotic
b. A monochorionic placenta is only seen with monozygotic twins
c. Chorionicity can be diagnosed on scan in >98% of pegnancies in the first trimester
d. Twin–twin transfusion syndrome is seen with monochorionic twins
e. Chorionicity not zygosity is an important determinant of risk with twin pregnancies

27 *Which of these is not usually associated with an increased risk of hyperemsis gravidarum?*

a. Molar pregnancy
b. Multiple pregnancy
c. Previous history of hyperemesis
d. First trimester of pregnancy
e. Increasing maternal age

28 *Which one of these is not an option for pain relief in the first stage of labour?*

a. TENS
b. Entonox
c. Epidural
d. Pudendal block
e. Morphine

29 *With which of these maternal infections is there no risk of intrapartum transmission to the fetus?*

a. Hepatitis B
b. HIV
c. *Chlamydia*
d. Hepatitis C
e. Rubella

30 *Which of the following help with prenatal screening for Down's syndrome?*

a. Maternal age
b. Fetal nuchal thickness
c. Mid-trimester maternal serum screening with bHCG and alpha-fetoprotein levels
d. Acetylcholinesterase estimation in the amniotic fluid
e. The integrated first and second trimester screening

EMQs

Obstetrics and Gynaecology: Clinical Cases Uncovered.
By M. Cruickshank and A. Shetty. Published 2009 by Blackwell
Publishing. ISBN 978-1-4051-8671-1.

1 Acute pelvic pain

a. Acute pelvic inflammatory disease
b. Ectopic pregnancy
c. Appendicitis
d. Torsion of ovarian cyst
e. Urinary tract infection
f. Miscarriage
g. Pancreatitis
h. Constipation
i. Endometriosis
j. Vulvovaginal thrush
k. Diverticulitis

The women below all presented with acute pelvic pain. Choose the most appropriate diagnosis from the above list.

1. A 25-year-old is admitted as an emergency with a 2-day history of right-sided lower abdominal pain and vomiting. On examination, she has a temperature of 37.5°C and a pulse of 86 beats/minute. She also has tenderness and guarding in her right iliac fossa. Her haemoglobin level is normal but she has a raised white blood cell count.

2. A 32-year-old presents with 36 hours of lower abdominal pain, dysuria and urinary frequency. She has a temperature of 38°C and her pulse is 78 beats/minute. She is slightly tender in her left loin.

3. A 26-year-old with a past history of *Chlamydia*, complains of right-sided lower abdominal pain, brown vaginal discharge and has a positive pregnancy test.

4. A 20-year-old complains of 3 days of lower abdominal pain and tenderness. On further questioning she admits to a yellow vaginal discharge. On examination, she looks slightly flushed and has a low grade pyrexia. She has lower abdominal tenderness and cervical excitation on examination. She has a raised white blood cell count and C-reactive protein (CRP).

5. A 30-year-old para 1 presents with cramping lower abdominal pain. She has heavy vaginal bleeding and notices fresh clots. Her last menstrual period (LMP) was 10 weeks ago and she has a positive pregnancy test.

6. A 24-year-old presents with 24 hours of right-sided abdominal pain. She describes the pain as colicky and today she vomited with the pain. She denies being sexually active and her LMP finished 3 days ago. On examination, she has tenderness and guarding in her right iliac fossa and bowel sounds are present. She has a raised white blood cell count. Ultrasound scan shows a 7 cm mass in the right adnexa.

2 Acute vulval pain

a. Syphilis
b. Vulval abscess
c. Bartholin's cyst
d. Herpes simplex
e. Sebaceous cyst
f. Bartholin's abscess
g. Vulval haematoma
h. Vulvovaginal thrush
i. Herpes zoster virus
j. Fixed drug eruption
k. Urethral caruncle

From the list of options given above, select the most likely diagnosis for each of the clinical scenarios given below. Each option may be used once, more than once or not at all.

1. A 30-year-old para 2 has a normal vaginal delivery at 39 weeks' gestation. Her first stage lasts 4 hours and the second stage lasts 4 minutes. She has active management of third stage and the midwife records that she has a small perineal abrasion which does not need suturing. Twelve hours later, she complains of severe vulval pain and discomfort. On examination, she has a large tense purple swelling distorting her right labia majora.

2. A 21-year-old para 0 returned from a holiday in Greece 5 days previously. She complains of intense vulval pain which has become increasingly severe over the last 24 hours. She thinks this may be caused by the chlorine in the hotel swimming pool. On examination, there is diffuse oedema, swelling and erythma with small blisters around the vaginal fourchette.

3. A 27-year-old para 0 complains of a 2-day history of throbbing vulva pain and tenderness on the left side of her vulva. She can no longer sit down because of a painful swelling to the left side of her posterior fourchette. On examination, there is a tense red swelling on the left side of the introitus which is too tender to allow further examination.

4. A 40-year-old woman with a 10-year history of type 1 diabetes gives a 2-day history of a painful swelling on her right labia majora. She had a previous episode which resolved when the swelling burst in a hot bath. On examination, she has an erythematous fluctuant swelling measuring 2 cm in diameter over her right labia majora.

5. A 59-year-old para 2 gives a 3-week history of vulval tenderness. She feels a very tender area 'inside' her vulva. The pain is worse on micturition. She last had a period at age 50 years and has never used hormone replacement therapy (HRT). On examination, there is a ring of polypoid tissue around the urethral meatus which is tender, red and pouting.

3 Contraception

a. Progestogen emergency contraception pills
b. Copper intrauterine device
c. Combined oral contraceptive pill
d. Vasectomy
e. Female laparoscopic clip sterilization
f. Progestogen contraceptive implant
g. Male latex condom
h. Female condom
i. Progestogen intrauterine system
j. Depot progestogen injection
k. Diaphragm

From the list of options given above, please select the most appropriate for the scenarios given below.

1. A couple both aged 39 have two children aged 16 and 14 years. They are certain that their family is complete. Both are healthy and she has no menstrual problems. Which would be their most effective contraceptive option.

2. An 18-year-old comes to the family planning clinic. She had sex 11 hours ago and is worried as her partner commented that the condom burst. On closer questioning she admits to another condom accident 8 days before. Her last period began 15 days ago. She should be offered this type of contraception initially.

3. A 35-year-old woman has two children aged 8 and 5 years. She is not sure if she wants a third child. She smokes 15 cigarettes a day. She is overweight (body mass index [BMI] 30) and is troubled by heavy but regular periods. This method of contraception would offer her most benefit.

4. A 35-year-old woman with no children and no current regular partner wishes to discuss contraception. She had a deep vein thrombosis after a long haul flight 2 years ago but no coagulopathy was diagnosed. This method of contraception is contraindicated for this woman.

5. A 22-year-old woman is happy with her progestogen implant for contraception. She has developed a latex allergy confirmed by patch testing. This additional method of barrier contraception could protect her from sexually transmitted infections.

4 Genitourinary medicine
a. *Candida*
b. Bacterial vaginosis
c. Cytomegalovirus
d. *Trichomonas vaginalis*
e. Gonorrhoea
f. Physiological discharge
g. Herpes simplex
h. Syphilis
i. Genital warts
j. *Chlamydia*
k. Herpes zoster

For each of the scenarios given above, select the most likely cause from the list of options.

1. An 18-year-old woman with a 4-month history of noticing several small rough lumps around the entrance to her vagina. She has no symptoms.
2. A 43-year-old woman who has noticed a watery 'fishy' smelling discharge which is often worse after a period. She has not been sexually active for 2 years and her last smear test was normal.
3. A 19-year-old woman has developed postcoital bleeding recently. She has a contraceptive implant fitted 2 years ago and her periods tend to be light and intermittent. She started a new sexual relationship 3 months ago.
4. A 14-year-old girl complains of vaginal discharge which marks her underwear. It is non-offensive and she has no itch or irritation. She notices that it is sometimes clear but sometimes slightly yellow and cloudy.
5. A 24-year-old woman develops several painful shallow ulcers on her labia minora and around the fourchette. She had sex with a casual partner 8 days ago.

5 Infertility
a. Hypothalamic ammenorrhoea
b. Polycystic ovarian syndrome
c. Turner's syndrome
d. Tubal factor infertility
e. Premature menopause
f. Oligospermia
g. Endometriosis
h. Hypothyroidism
i. Unexplained infertility
j. Type 1 diabetes
k. Hyperthyroidism

For each of the following couples who present for the investigation of subfertility, select the single most likely diagnosis from the list of options given above.

1. A 29-year-old woman with a history of irregular bleeding and increased BMI (36) presents with a 2-year history of primary infertility. Her partner's semen analysis is normal.
2. A 25-year-old athlete presents with secondary amenorrhoea for 6 months and primary infertility. Her BMI is 18. Her partner's semen analysis is normal.
3. A 32-year-old woman presents with a 2-year history of primary infertility. She stopped the combined oral contraceptive pill 2 years ago. Since then she has experienced very heavy and painful but regular periods. She also complains of deep dysparunia. Her partner's semen analysis is normal.
4. A 28-year-old women presents with an 18-month history of primary infertility and dull lower abdominal pain. She has regular menstrual cycles and her partner's semen analysis is normal. She was diagnosed with *Chlamydia* 5 years previously and following a course of doxycycline her *Chlamydia* test was negative.

> **6 Therapeutic options for specific indications in pregnancy**
> 1. Syntometrine
> 2. Oxytocin
> 3. Benzyl penicillin
> 4. Erythromycin
> 5. Vaginal prostaglandin E_2
> 6. Atosiban
> 7. Folic acid
> 8. Magnesium sulphate
> 9. 0.9% normal saline infusion
> 10. Prophylactic dalteparin

For the list of therapeutic options given above, select the single most appropriate clinical condition below. Each option may be used once, more than once, or not at all.

a. A 23-year-old para 2 with confirmed prelabour rupture of membranes at 30 weeks' gestation and no signs of chorioamnionitis or fetal concerns.

b. A 20-year-old para 1 who presents at 30 weeks' gestation with three moderate uterine contractions every 10 minutes. Her cervical assessment shows her to be in early labour with the cervix being 3 cm dilated and 50% effaced. You wish to administer steroids for fetal lung maturity

c. A 36-year-old para 3 who has been well antenatally and intrapartum, has a spontaneous vaginal delivery at term. Following delivery of the placenta there is a 500 mL vaginal blood loss and the uterus feels a little boggy. The placenta is checked and looks complete.

d. A primipara has her labour induced at 39 +3 weeks' gestation for the indication of pre-eclampsia and a growth restricted baby. Her cervix is favourable and she has an artificial rupture of membranes. There is no uterine activity.

e. An induction of labour is planned for a primipara at 38 weeks' gestation for the indication of cholestasis of pregnancy. Her cervical Bishop's score is 4.

f. A 32-year-old para 2 is admitted with hyperemesis gravidarum at 12 weeks' gestation. She has +++ ketonuria.

g. A 40-year-old para 2 (two previous caesarean sections) has her third planned caesarean section at 39 weeks' gestation. She has a BMI of 39 and is a smoker.

h. A 26-year-old woman on carbamazepine for control of epilepsy is seen for prepregnancy counselling. Her epilepsy is under good control and she is hoping to come off contraception and try for a pregnancy soon.

i. A 33-year-old primipara is in spontaneous labour at 41 +2 weeks' gestation. Her cervix is 4 cm dilated, fully effaced, membranes are intact and she is having moderately strong uterine contractions about 3–4 every 10 minutes. A urine culture at 15 weeks' gestation had grown group B streptococci.

j. An 18-year-old primigravida is in hospital at 35 weeks' gestation for pre-eclampsia (BP 150/94 mmHg, +++ proteinuria). She is now complaining of pain in her epigastrium and is asking for paracetamol for a headache. Her reflexes are brisk with clonus.

> **7 Antenatal tests on mother and fetus**
> 1. Nuchal translucency (NT) measurement in the first trimester
> 2. Mid-trimester anomaly ultrasound scan
> 3. Alpha-fetoprotein elevated on mid-trimester serum screening
> 4. Urine for proteinuria
> 5. Amniocentesis
> 6. External cephalic version
> 7. Screening for sickle cell
> 8. Doppler scan of umbilical blood flow
> 9. Cardiotocogram (CTG)
> 10. Mid-stream sample of urine for culture

Match the antenatal test/intervention given in the list above to the most appropriate option below. Each option may be used once, more than once or not at all.

a. Reduced fetal movements for 24 hours at 37 weeks' gestation

b. A fetal growth scan at 32 weeks' gestation showing abdominal circumference below the 5th centile and reduced liquor volume

c. Dysuria and suprapubic discomfort at 24 weeks' gestation

d. Spina bifida in the fetus

e. Screening test for Down's syndrome

f. Screening for gestational diabetes

g. Diagnostic test for Down's syndrome

h. Diagnostic test for chorioamnionitis

i. Breech presentation at 37 weeks' gestation

j. Routine antenatal check at 28 weeks' gestation

k. An 18-year-old Nigerian woman booking at 11 weeks' gestation

l. Cleft lip in the fetus

> **8 Complications associated with pregnancy and their clinical presentation**
> 1. Placenta praevia
> 2. Twin–twin transfusion syndrome
> 3. Chorioamnionitis
> 4. Scar rupture
> 5. Placental abruption
> 6. Cord prolapse
> 7. Preterm labour
> 8. Pyelonephritis
> 9. HELLP syndrome
> 10. Endometritis

Match the diagnoses given above to the single most likely clinical scenario given below. Each option may be used once, more than once, or not at all.

a. A 16-year-old primigravida complains of some blurred vision and epigastric pain at 31 weeks' gestation. Her blood pressure is 140/90 mmHg and there is ++++ proteinuria. Her blood results include: haemoglobin 9 g/dL, low platelet count 95×10^9/L, increased serum urate 0.40 nmol/L and alanine aminotransferase 186 IU/L, normal serum bilirubin 10 IU/L, urea 5 nmol/L.

b. A 22-year-old para 0 has symptoms of nausea, vomiting, fever and back pain at 36 weeks' gestation. On examination, she looks flushed and dehydrated with a temperature of 38.5 °C and she has right-sided renal angle tenderness. Her uterus is soft and non-tender and she is feeling good fetal movements.

c. A para 0 has about 200 mL of fresh painless vaginal bleeding at 34 weeks' gestation. The baby is in an oblique beech position with a normal CTG tracing.

d. A para 1 at 28 weeks' gestation complains of abdominal pain and small amount of fresh vaginal bleeding. Her uterus is contracting about 6 in 10 minutes, there is not much uterine relaxation between contractions and there is fetal tachycardia, reduced baseline variability and late decelerations on the CTG.

e. A para 4, with a history of insulin-dependent diabetes, has been admitted to the ward with polyhydramnios and an unstable lie of the fetus at 37 weeks' gestation. On her way to the toilet she feels a sudden large gush of fluid per vaginum. She gets back to her bed and presses the emergency buzzer. When the midwife checks her the uterus is soft, non-tender, with no uterine contractions and the fetal heart is found to be 60 beats/minute.

f. A 27-year-old para 1 has a secondary postpartum haemorrhage (PPH) of 800 mL, 10 days after delivery. Her temperature is 37.8 °C, she has some tenderness in her lower abdomen, but no guarding or rigidity, and her uterus seems to be involuting. On vaginal examination, the cervical os closed and there is some tenderness over the uterus.

g. A 33-year-old is being managed conservatively following confirmed prelabour rupture of membranes at 30 weeks' gestation. At admission her CRP is <10 and white blood cell count 9×10^9/L. At 31 +2 weeks, her CRP is noted to be at 60 and white blood cell count 18.8×10^9/L. On examination, she is found to be slightly tender over the uterus and there is a fetal tachycardia of 180 beats/minute.

h. A 30-year-old with monochorionic twins is scanned at 22 weeks' gestation. She complains of a sudden increase in her abdominal girth. One twin is noted to have its abdominal circumference at the 10th centile with 2 cm pools of liquor, with the other twin at the 90th centile with 9 cm pools of liquor.

i. A 19-year-old para 0 at 32 weeks' gestation, on antibiotics for a confirmed urinary tract infection, complains of abdominal tightenings every 3–4 minutes with a mucosy discharge per vaginum. The midwife examines her and finds her cervix to be 1 cm long and 3.5 cm dilated.

j. A 33-year-old para 1 (previous caesarean section) is having a trial of vaginal birth. She makes good progress until 5 cm dilatation, when she complains of a continuous pain in the suprapubic area. The midwife notices fresh bleeding per vaginum and there are decelerations on the CTG.

k. A 28-year-old para 0 presents with postcoital painless spotting of blood per vaginum at 35 weeks. The fetal head is fixed in the pelvis, her uterus is soft with a normal fetal heart rate. Following a scan, a speculum examination is performed which shows a cervical ectropion, with no further bleeding seen.

9 Clinical features and their associations

1. BP, urine protein
2. Symphysiofundal height
3. Increasing maternal age
4. Intrauterine fetal growth restriction
5. Bicornuate uterus
6. Grand multiparity
7. Fetal macrosomia
8. Folic acid periconception
9. Hyperemesis gravidarum
10. Previous caesarean section

From the list above, which would be the single most appropriate association from the options below? Each option may be used once, more than once, or not at all.

a. Prevention of fetal neural tube defects
b. Screening for fetal growth problems
c. Smoking
d. Molar pregnancy
e. Pregnancy in an insulin-dependent diabetic woman
f. Atonic PPH
g. Increased risk of gastroschisis
h. Preterm labour
i. Screening for pre-eclampsia
j. Increasing incidence of trisomy 21
k. Low lying or adherent placenta

10 Indications for interventions in pregnancy

1. Elective caesarean section for delivery
2. Maternal immunization postpartum
3. Neonatal immunization
4. Anti D administration in a rhesus negative mother
5. Betamethasone for fetal lung maturity
6. Vitamin B_{12} supplementation
7. Hydralazine infusion
8. Continuous CTG monitoring
9. Syntometrine
10. Higher (5 mg) dose of periconception folic acid

From the list above, select the single most appropriate association for the options below. Each option may be used once, more than once, or not at all.

a. Mean arterial pressure of 134 in a para 0 in labour with pre-eclampsia.
b. Fresh thick meconium seen in labour.
c. Severe hyperemesis gravidarum.
d. Insulin-dependent diabetes mellitus.
e. Mother diagnosed to have chronic hepatitis B on antenatal screening.
f. Para 2 with previous history of atonic PPH now in the third stage of labour.
g. Amniocentesis performed at 16 weeks' gestation.
h. Mother non-immune to rubella on antenatal screening.
i. HIV positive mother on HAART with a viral load of 10100 at 37 weeks.
j. Mother diagnosed to be hepatitis C positive on antenatal screening.
k. Prelabour preterm rupture of membranes at 28 weeks' gestation.
l. A primipara with non-progress of labour.

SAQs

1 *A 75-year-old woman presents with vague abdominal symptoms. She is unmarried and has no children. Over the past 2 months she has noticed that her abdomen seems to be swollen and she cannot fasten the button in her waistbands. She last had a period at age 50 years and has had no vaginal bleeding since. Her bowels move regularly and an faecal occult blood test is negative. On examination, she has a distended abdomen with noticeable shifting dullness and a fluid thrill.*

a. List three initial investigations that you would perform to help you to establish the most likely diagnosis? *(3 marks)*
b. Why are these investigations important in determining her future management? *(2 marks)*
c. The investigations reveal that advanced ovarian cancer is the most likely diagnosis and a laparotomy is planned. What are the aims of surgery in this situation? *(4 marks)*
d. This diagnosis is confirmed. What type of adjuvant treatment do you need to consider? *(2 marks)*
e. If she was found to have bilateral pleural effusions and cytological examination of the fluid taken by a pleural tap identified adenocarcinoma cells, what would this additional information mean for her prognosis? *(2 marks)*

2 *Veronica is a 53-year-old cleaner. She had three normal vaginal deliveries in her twenties. Her periods stopped 5 years ago. She now complains of increasing incontinence of urine while laughing, coughing and running. She also mentions that she has some intermittent urinary urgency. She consults her GP about this problem.*

a. Suggest six relevant questions that you might ask Veronica to find out more about her presenting complaint? *(Up to maximum of 6 marks)*
On clinical abdominal examination, your findings are normal. On vaginal examination, the anterior vaginal wall is bulging and visible prior to inserting a Sims speculum. Her uterus and posterior vaginal wall are well supported.
b. What is your diagnosis? *(2 marks)*
c. What test would you arrange for next? *(1 mark)*
d. Suggest four conservative measures that you could suggest at the clinic to improve her symptoms. *(4 marks)*
Veronica feels distressed by her symptoms as she works as a cleaner and she feels that it restricts what she is able to do. She has told her employer that she cannot do heavy work because of 'back problems' as she is embarrassed to reveal her difficulties.
e. What further treatment could you consider? *(2 marks)*
Veronica decides to have non-surgical treatment. She finds the incontinence is still present, but the lump has disappeared. She tried physiotherapy exercises but they have not improved her situation and she is getting more depressed.
f. What investigation would you consider and why? *(2 marks)*

Obstetrics and Gynaecology: Clinical Cases Uncovered.
By M. Cruickshank and A. Shetty. Published 2009 by Blackwell Publishing. ISBN 978-1-4051-8671-1.

3 *A 45-year-old woman, G3 P3, has been referred to the gynaecology outpatient clinic with a history of heavy periods. She has been using tranexamic acid as recommended by her GP, but has not noticed any improvement in her symptoms. She has no past medical history of note and she is a schoolteacher. There were no abnormal findings on examination of the abdomen and pelvis.*

a. What are three differential diagnoses that come to mind? *(3 marks)*
b. List six questions you ask when taking her menstrual history. *(6 marks)*
c. Name three investigations you would consider to assist in making a diagnosis. *(3 marks)*
   All further investigations are normal.
d. Name two other medical treatment options available to this patient, and give one side-effect of each. *(4 marks)*
   This patient is unwilling to try any other form of medical treatment. She would like to discuss surgical options.
e. What would you suggest to her as a reasonable surgical option? Justify your choice of surgical treatment and give two side-effects of this option. *(5 marks)*
f. Name three different ways in which a hysterectomy can be performed? *(3 marks)*
g. In the case of women with high BMI, what other specialty would you consult with prior to undertaking any surgical intervention? *(1 mark)*

4 *A 20-year-old girl presents with fresh vaginal bleeding. Her LMP was 6 weeks ago. She uses condoms for contraception.*

a. List four features in history that will aid diagnosis. *(4 marks)*
b. What four features would you look for on examination? *(4 marks)*
c. What four non-imaging investigations would you consider to aid you with the diagnosis and management of this patient? *(4 marks)*
d. What imaging investigation would you request to assist you in the management of this patient? *(2 marks)*

5 *Mrs Ross is a 72-year-old widow who presents with a painful ulcer on her left labia majora. She also reports noticing some bloodstained spots on her underwear. She has suffered from vulva itch for the last 5 years. The itch is worse at night and none of the creams bought at her local pharmacy have helped. She tried a steroid cream prescribed by her GP with no benefit. She thinks that she may have damaged her skin by scratching it. On examination, she has a raised grey plaque of slightly nodular skin involving most of her perineum with a central area of irregular deep ulceration.*

a. What is the most likely diagnosis? *(2 marks)*
b. Name three underlying aetiological factors that may predispose to the development of this condition. *(6 marks)*
c. Which investigation should you perform? *(2 marks)*
d. Her biopsy excludes malignancy. What is your next course of action and why? *(3 marks)*

6 *Mrs Neale, a primigravida, arrives on the labour ward at 41 weeks +3 days' gestation. She thinks her labour has started. She has a mucosy 'show' but no leak of fluid per vaginum. Her uterine contractions were infrequent some hours ago, but have become more regular and painful over the last 2 hours. The frequency of these contractions is about three every 10 minutes, with each lasting for about 50 seconds. The fetal heart rate is regular at around 140 beats/minute. On examination, her cervix is found to be fully effaced and 4 cm dilated, membranes are intact and the fetal head is at −1 station.*

a. (i) Is Mrs Neale in active labour? *(1 mark)* (ii) What are the reasons to support your diagnosis? *(2 marks)*
   She requests pain relief.
b. Name four suitable options she could be offered at this time. *(4 marks)*
   Three hours later her membranes rupture and the liquor is noted to be meconium stained.
c. (i) What might be the significance of this meconium? *(2 marks)* (ii) List one non-interventional measure you could undertake to determine fetal well-being. *(1 mark)*
   The fetal condition is shown to be fine. Her contractions are now about two every 10 minutes and mild to moderate in intensity. On a vaginal examination, 4 hours after the last one, cervical dilation is 4.5 cm.

d. (i) What do you conclude from this assessment? *(1 mark)* (ii) What is your next action? *(2 marks)*

> **7** *A midwife refers a 20-year-old primigravida with a history of 9 weeks' amenorrhoea and vomiting over the past 2 weeks which has worsened over the last 2 days, with inability to keep any fluids down.*

a. What symptoms would you wish to ask her about (list three)? *(3 marks)*
b. What clinical signs would you look for to aid diagnosis (list three)? *(3 marks)*
c. List at least three investigations you would wish to do. *(6 marks)*
d. What would your management plan include? *(6 marks)*
e. Apart from hyperemesis gravidarum, what can cause vomiting in pregnancy (list two)? *(2 marks)*

> **8** *An 18-year-old para 0 is sent in to the day assessment unit by her midwife at 36 weeks' gestation when she was noted to have a blood pressure of 150/98 mmHg and +++ proteinuria at a routine check. Her booking BP had been 110/70 mmHg.*

a. What particular symptoms would you wish to ask her about (list five)? *(5 marks)*
b. Knowing her blood pressure to now be 160/110 mmHg with +++ proteinuria, what would you look for on examination (list three)? *(3 marks)*
c. She complains of a headache and her reflexes are seen to be brisk with clonus 3 beats. What does her clinical condition indicate? *(1 mark)*
d. What would the management include? *(6 marks)*

> **9** *A para 2 at 37 weeks' gestation is referred by her midwife to the antenatal clinic as she thinks the baby might be in an oblique breech lie. You confirm the lie on abdominal palpation. She has had two previous vaginal deliveries and has no significant medical or obstetric history of note.*

a. What investigation would you arrange for and what would you be looking for with this? *(2 marks)*
b. What would you advise and why? *(2 marks)*
c. What would you discuss about the procedure? *(4 marks)*

---

d. Give two causes for/associations with fetal malposition. *(2 marks)*

> **10** *Mrs Smith, a 39-year-old para 0 books into the antenatal clinic at 11 weeks' gestation. She has no particular medical history of note.*

a. She wishes to discuss the tests that she could consider for screening for Down's syndrome. What options would you discuss with her? *(6 marks)*
b. Because of the false negative results that may occur with the screening tests, she opts for a diagnostic test based on her age-related risk of Down's syndrome. What would you discuss with her? *(4 marks)*
c. She asks what other routine screening tests would be offered to her at booking. *(5 marks)*

1. e	11. d	21. b
2. d	12. c	22. a
3. a	13. a	23. b
4. a	14. d	24. b
5. c	15. d	25. b
6. c	16. b	26. a
7. d	17. e	27. e
8. b	18. d	28. d
9. a	19. c	29. e
10. d	20. c	30. d

Obstetrics and Gynaecology: Clinical Cases Uncovered.
By M. Cruickshank and A. Shetty. Published 2009 by Blackwell
Publishing. ISBN 978-1-4051-8671-1.

EMQs answers

1
1. c
2. e
3. b
4. a
5. f
6. d

2
1. g
2. d
3. f
4. b
5. k

3
1. d
2. b
3. i
4. c
5. h

4
1. i
2. b
3. j
4. f
5. g

5
1. b
2. a

3. g
4. d

6
1. c
2. d
3. i
4. a
5. e
6. b
7. h
8. j
9. f
10. g

7
1. e
2. l
3. d
4. j
5. g
6. i
7. k
8. b
9. a
10. c

8
1. c
2. h
3. g
4. j

5. d
6. e
7. i
8. b
9. a
10. f

9
1. i
2. b
3. j
4. c
5. h
6. f
7. e
8. a, e
9. d
10. k

10
1. i
2. h
3. e
4. g
5. k
6. c
7. a
8. b
9. f
10. d

Obstetrics and Gynaecology: Clinical Cases Uncovered.
By M. Cruickshank and A. Shetty. Published 2009 by Blackwell
Publishing. ISBN 978-1-4051-8671-1.

SAQs answers

1 Pelvic mass

a. Serum CA125
   Ultrasound scan of abdomen and pelvis
   CT scan of abdomen and pelvis
   Ascitic tap for cytology
   (3 marks)

b. The results will be used to calculate her risk of malignancy index. If this is raised she needs to be referred urgently to a gynaecology oncologist
   (2 marks)

c. Obtain tissue for histological diagnosis
   Debulk tumour as much as possible
   Relieve symptoms, e.g. from pressure or bowel obstruction
   Perform total abdominal hysterectomy and bilateral salpingo-oopherectomy (TAH/BSO)/omentectomy/peritoneal washing
   (4 marks)

d. Chemotherapy. Platinum as a single agent or in combination with taxol *(2 marks)*

e. Positive cytology from pleural fluid means she has stage 4 disease and the 5-year survival is less than 5% *(2 marks)*

2 Prolapse

a. (i) Other urinary symptoms that she has not mentioned to complete your history
   • Nocturia (getting up once at night is considered normal)
   • Dysuria or haematuria (you need to consider urinary tract infection [UTI])
   • Urinary frequency (4–6 times per day is considered normal)
   • Urge incontinence (as she has only mentioned urgency)

• Voiding problems (e.g. she may have difficulty initiating micturition or need to double void, she may need to push her prolapses back to void)
• Degree of incontinence (does she need to wear pads or change her clothes, how much urine does she lose, how often is she wet?)
(ii) Any lump felt or seen vaginally (prolapse)
(iii) Is she on hormone replacement therapy (HRT) and what type?
(iv) Cough or chest symptoms/asthma/smoking
     Weight gain/BMI
     Ask her if she works and what job she does.
       Does it involve lifting or other stress?
(v) It is important to know if her symptoms affect her work or other usual activities such as hobbies and sexual function
(vi) Difficult labour or prolonged second stage
     Large babies
(6 marks)

b. Cytocoele and stress incontinence. This provisional diagnosis has been made from her history and the findings of cystocoele on examination *(2 marks)*

c. Mid-stream specimen of urine (MSSU). It is important to exclude UTI in any women with urinary symptoms *(1 mark)*

d. Weight loss (increased pressure on the pelvic floor will exacerbate her problems)
   Advice on how to stop smoking
   Pelvic floor exercises with bladder retraining (these are recommended as a combined approach for women with urinary incontinence)
   Practice double voiding
   (4 marks)

e. Ring pessary
   Surgery
   (2 marks)

f. Cystometry may be useful to identify if the incontinence is caused by detrusor overactivity or urethral sphincter weakness. This will identify those

Obstetrics and Gynaecology: Clinical Cases Uncovered.
By M. Cruickshank and A. Shetty. Published 2009 by Blackwell Publishing. ISBN 978-1-4051-8671-1.

women who require a suburethral taping (e.g.tension free vaginal tape by transvaginal or obturator route) for their stress incontinence. *(2 marks)*

3 Heavy menstrual bleeding

a. Dysfunctional uterine bleeding
Endometrial polyp
Endometrial hyperplasia
Endometriosis
Adenomyosis
Endometrial cancer (uncommon in this age group)
(1 mark per item to a maximum of 3)
b. Number of days of bleeding
Duration of cycle
Abnormal bleeding (intermenstrual bleeding, postcoital bleeding)
How many pads or tampons she uses
Flooding
Clots
Effect of bleeding on lifestyle
Use of contraception
Last cervical smear test
Menarche
(1 mark per item to a maximum of 6)
c. Ultrasound scan
Endometrial biopsy
Hysteroscopy
Full blood count
Ultrasound scan may reveal endometrial polyps or fibroids
An endometrial biopsy can show hyperplasia or atypia and can rule out malignancy
Hysteroscopy will enable visualization of the endometrial cavity and can diagnose endometrial polyps, submucosal fibroids and endometrial cancer
A full blood count (FBC) can be helpful in cases of iron deficiency anaemia secondary to heavy menstrual bleeding
D&C would not be accepted as an answer as it is an outdated investigation
Thyroid function tests are not useful unless the patient has symptoms suggestive of a thyroid disorder
(1 mark per item to a maximum of 3)
d. NSAIDs (e.g. mefenamic acid) should be considered as first line treatment along with tranexamic acid which she has already tried (side-effects: indigestion, diarrhoea, vomiting, aggravation of peptic ulcer disease)

Mirena IUS is very effective and in this patient could be left in place until she reaches the menopause (side-effects: irregular spotting, bleeding, breast tenderness, acne, headaches, small risk of uterine perforation at insertion)
Combined oral contraceptive (COC) pill (side-effects: breast tenderness, nausea, mood changes, rarely, deep vein thrombosis). COC may be considered in younger age groups but this patient is aged 45 years
(2 marks each, i.e. 1 for method and 1 for side-effect)
e. Endometrial ablation:
Less invasive
Less surgical risk
Fast recovery
Day case procedure
Completed family
Side-effects:
Vaginal discharge
Pelvic pain
Infection
Uterine perforation
May need additional surgery, procedure failure
(2 marks for choosing endometrial ablation, 1 for any of the factors to justify this and 2 for side-effects)
Hysterectomy: (not first choice)
Completed family
Patient may want to be completely free of having periods
Side-effects: intraoperative or postoperative haemorrhage, infection (UTI, wound), damage to bowel or bladder at operation, deep vein thrombosis, pulmonary embolus
(1 mark for choosing hysterectomy, 1 for any of the factors to justify this and 2 for side-effects)
f. Abdominal hysterectomy
Vaginal hysterectomy
Laparoscopic-assisted vaginal hysterectomy
Total laparoscopic hysterectomy
(1 mark per item to a maximum of 3)
g. Anaesthetic review is important in obese patients before deciding on surgery *(1 mark)*

4 Bleeding in early pregnancy

a. Amount of bleeding
(i) Length of menstrual cycles
(ii) Associated pain
(iii) History of pelvic inflammatory disease/ appendicectomy/previous ectopic pregnancy

You should suspect from the history that she has bleeding in early pregnancy and you need to assess the severity of her bleeding, the duration of amenorrhoea and gestation (based on her normal cycle length) and if there are any features that would increase her risk of ectopic pregnancy. *(4 marks)*

b. (i) Pulse rate
(ii) Blood pressure
(iii) Abdominal tenderness
(iv) Speculum examination to look at cervical os
You need to assess her clinical state because she is actively bleeding. Tenderness suggests an ectopic pregnancy. Examination of the cervical os will confirm if a miscarriage is inevitable. *(4 marks)*

c. (i) Urinary pregnancy test
(ii) Urine dipstick
(iii) FBC
(iv) Serum β human chorionic gonadotrophin (HCG)
(4 marks)

d. Ultrasound of the pelvis. This will identify if she has an intrauterine pregnancy and if it is viable. If the uterus is empty, you need to consider this along with the result of the serum βHCG and your clinical findings *(2 marks)*

5 Vulval pain

a. Squamous cell cancer of the vulva. The clinical findings suggest vulval intraepithelial neoplasia (VIN) with an area which has progressed to a squamous cell cancer of the vulva. The brief clinical scenario of itch not relieved by any topical treatments also suggests VIN although this can be a feature of lichen sclerosus *(2 marks)*

b. VIN
Lichen sclerosus
Lichen planus
(6 marks)

c. She needs a diagnostic skin biopsy. This is to confirm the diagnosis and to determine if there is any evidence of invasion. This can be performed under local anaesthetic but you need to ensure that the biopsy is of sufficient size and depth and the most suspicious area is biopsied. As invasion is suspected clinically, you should not perform an excision biopsy as this may compromise further surgery if it turns out to be a cancer. *(2 marks)*

d. She needs to have the area excised to ensure that there is no invasion in the residual areas. If there is only VIN, this will also provide her with symptom relief. In this older age group and with a single lesion, the risk of recurrence is low (compared to younger women with multifocal disease) but she should be seen for follow-up *(3 marks)*

6 Labour

a. (i) Yes *(1 mark)*
(ii) Her cervix is fully effaced and dilating *(1 mark)*
Her contractions are getting regular and increasing in intensity and frequency *(1 mark)*

b. TENS *(1 mark)*
Birthing pool *(1 mark)*
Morphine/pethidine *(1 mark)*
Nitrous oxide (Entonox) inhalation *(1 mark)*
Epidural block *(1 mark)*

c. (i) Could mean fetal distress or hypoxia *(1 mark)*
May be a result of fetal postmaturity *(1 mark)*
(ii) Continuous fetal cardiotocograph (CTG) *(1 mark)*

d. (i) Poor or inadequate progress of labour *(1 mark)* *or* inco-ordinate uterine activity *(1 mark)*
(ii) Augmentation of labour with a carefully titrated oxytocin intravenous infusion *(2 marks)*

7 Hyperemesis

a. Abdominal pain, heartburn *(1 mark)*
Urinary symptoms – dysuria, frequency, haematuria, urine volumes *(1 mark)*
Diarrhoea *(1 mark)*
Fever *(1 mark)*
Jaundice *(1 mark)*
Trigger factors for vomiting, duration, frequency *(1 mark)*

b. Pulse, BP (may be tachycardic, or have postural hypotension) *(1 mark)*
Temperature *(1 mark)*
Signs of dehydration – decreased skin turgor, dry skin, mouth, eyes *(1 mark)*
Icterus

c. Urinalysis for ketones, leucocytes, nitrites, MSSU for culture/sensitivity (+ for urine pregnancy test if not already confirmed) *(2 marks)*
Bloods for FBC, urea and electrolytes, liver function tests, thyroid function tests *(2 marks)*

Pelvic ultrasound to confirm viable pregnancy (singleton or multiple) and rule out molar pregnancy *(2 marks)*

d. Commence intravenous fluids (*not* 5% dextrose) – at least 3 L/day with electrolyte management as required (e.g. for hyponatraemia, hypokalaemia) *(2 marks)*

Regular antiemetics – e.g. promethazine, metaclopramide, cyclizine *(1 mark)*

Strict intake/output fluid chart with regular checks for ketonuria (2–3 times a day) *(1 mark)*

Pulse/BP/temperature chart 4-hourly *(1 mark)*

Consider thrombophylaxis *(1 mark)*

Thiamine replacement *(1 mark)*

e. Pylenephritis/UTI *(1 mark)*

Gastroenteritis *(1 mark)*

Hepatitis *(1 mark)*

Pancreatitis *(1 mark)*

Appendicitis *(1 mark)*

8 Pre-eclampsia

a. Headaches

Visual disturbance

Upper abdominal/epigastric pain

Nausea, vomiting

Increase in swelling (legs, rings getting tighter)

Urine output volumes (normal or reduced)

Has she been feeling good fetal movements?

(1 mark each)

b. Epigastric/right hypochondrial tenderness (over the liver)

Brisk reflexes/clonus

Significant peripheral swelling

Papilloedema on fundoscopy

(1 mark each)

c. She has severe pre-eclampsia and is at risk of its complications especially of convulsions/eclampsia and those associated with high blood pressure (e.g. intracranial haemorrhage) *(1 mark)*

d. IV cannula/blood samples for urgent FBC (including platelet count), serum urate, urea and electrolytes, liver function tests, group and save

Check fetal heart (CTG)

Hydralazine for control of blood pressure

Magnesium sulphate for prophylaxis against eclampsia

Transfer to high risk setting on labour ward for intensive monitoring (BP, pulse, respiration, neurological state, intake output chart)

Depending on further clinical condition, blood results and state of her cervix, plan for induction of labour or caesarean section once acute condition is under control

(1 mark each)

9 Fetal malposition

a. Ultrasound scan – look for placental position (whether low lying), confirm lie of the fetus, liquor volume (especially for polyhydramnios) *(2 marks)*

b. As she is at term with the baby in an oblique position, it is advisable she stays in hospital as an inpatient because of the risk of rupture of membranes with the cord prolapsing. Cord prolapse would necessitate an emergency delivery because of the associated acute fetal risks *(1 mark)*

The option of external cephalic version (ECV) should be discussed with her once the scan has ruled out anything of concern *(1 mark)*

c. It involves external manipulation of the baby through the maternal abdomen to turn the baby to a cephalic position *(1 mark)*

Uterine tocolysis is recommended as it improves the success of the procedure *(1 mark)*

The success rate is about 60% in parous women, and there is a <5% chance that the baby will turn back again to a malposition after a successful ECV *(1 mark)*

The (uncommon) risks of the procedure include spontaneous rupture of membranes, retroplacental haemorrhage and cord accidents which may lead to fetal concerns necessitating emergency delivery *(1 mark)*

d. Low lying placenta

Polyhydramnios

Uterine abnormality, fibroids in the lower segment

Grand multiparity

(1 mark each)

10 Antenatal screening for Down's syndrome

a. Based on her age alone (trisomy 21 has an increasing incidence with age), her risk would be approximately 1:100 (at age 40 at delivery) *(1 mark)*

Between 11 and 14 weeks: age + nuchal thickness alone or in combination with βHCG and PAPP-A levels in maternal serum *(1 mark)*

Between 14 and 20 weeks: mid-trimester triple or quadruple test on serum screening (age + βHCG + alpha-fetoprotein + unconjugated estriol + inhibin A) *(1 mark)*

11–14 weeks+: 14–20 weeks screening – the integrated test *(1 mark)*

All these tests have false positive and false negative rates. If the results come back with a high risk of trisomy 21, a diagnostic test would be recommended to check the fetal karytotype *(2 marks)*

b. The diagnostic tests available include chorionic villus sampling (CVS) which is usually performed between 10 and 14 weeks. It carries a 2% risk of miscarriage *(2 marks)*

Amniocentesis is performed from 15 weeks' gestation, it carries a 1% risk of procedure-related pregnancy loss *(2 marks)*

There is also a small (1%) risk of failed culture, and mosaicism (particularly with CVS) which may require repeat testing

c. FBC

Blood group, rhesus status and red cell antibodies

Immunity status to rubella

Screening for hepatitis B infection

Screening for HIV infection

Screening for syphilis infection

Urine for MSSU for asymptomatic bacteruria

(1 mark each)

Index of cases by diagnosis

Index

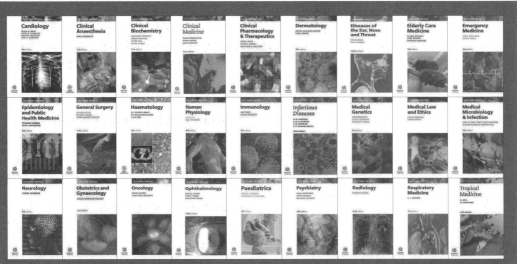
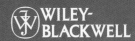

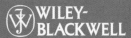